John G. Bruhn

After Diagnosis: Family Caregiving with Hospice Patients

Springer

John G. Bruhn
Department of Sociology
Northern Arizona University
Flagstaff, AZ
USA

ISSN 2211-7644 ISSN 2211-7652 (electronic)
SpringerBriefs in Well-Being and Quality of Life Research
ISBN 978-3-319-29801-6 ISBN 978-3-319-29803-0 (eBook)
DOI 10.1007/978-3-319-29803-0

Library of Congress Control Number: 2016931842

Printed on acid-free paper

This Springer imprint is published by SpringerNature
The registered company is Springer International Publishing AG Switzerland

SpringerBriefs in Well-Being and Quality of Life Research

More information about this series at http://www.springer.com/series/10150

To the hospice patients
who inspire others to live
hopefully and to die courageously

Old friends pass away, new friends appear. It is just like the days.
An old day passes, a new day arrives.
The important thing is to make it meaningful:
a meaningful friend – or a meaningful day.

—Dalai Lama

There is a light in this world, a healing spirit more powerful than any darkness we may encounter. We sometimes lose sight of this force when there is suffering, and too much pain. Then suddenly, the spirit will emerge through the lives of ordinary people who hear a call and answer in extraordinary ways.

—Mother Teresa

Acknowledgments

Hospice provided me with the opportunity to participate as a volunteer respite caregiver over the past 10 years. Periodic workshops and peer-group gatherings enabled volunteers to share experiences, gain support from each other, and become advocates for hospice as an excellent option for terminal care.

Tracy Grindle typed numerous drafts of this book and provided valued suggestions. Vince Colburn contributed his excellent skills in graphic art.

A Note to Readers

All of the patient examples and narratives are real, but details regarding demographics and social and psychological factors have been altered to protect patient privacy and identity. The patients were assigned to me for respite care until they passed. I did not interview patients or use a standard questionnaire or a recording device. My data was primarily based on my observation and interaction with family members. This is a book of reflective learning and is not intended to be a formal, scientific study. I was "with" patients for an average of two to four hours weekly for about six months. My role was as a respite volunteer who enabled the caregiver to experience unstructured time (respite).

Contents

Introduction

The image some people have of dying is a hopeless, helpless, lonely, and often painful ordeal that creates a financial, emotional, and caregiving burden on the family (Leary 2012). Other people, with the help of guided imagery, have a less threatening view of dying and death (Staudt and Ellens 2013). It seems that we all hope for "a good death"—sudden, painless, and with no or limited imposition on others.

In reality, dying is a lifelong process that begins with birth (Kastenbaum 2002). Dying is a part of living. We have choices in how we want to live life and, to some extent, how we want to die. Our attitudes toward living also influence our attitudes towards death. It is not unexpected that as we age we will have to live with the consequences of a disabling chronic disease. Some diseases impose significant limitations in how we can live life, others have minimal limitations. We can't select our diseases, they pick us, but we can choose how we live and die with them. Ultimately we all die from the same cause—our hearts stop. It is what is in our hearts that make us different, and how we connect with the hearts of others that determines our legacy.

The process of dying is unique to each individual and family. At one extreme, individuals share few, if any, of their thoughts and feelings about dying. At the other extreme, individuals wish to complete unfinished business and plan their own funerals. Between those extremes, people express a variety of feelings as their physical and mental conditions change. Families and friends may help or hinder the dying process with their own agendas. The dying process is often difficult for the survivors as they waver about what to do, or not to do, in their projections of what they think should be "a good death" for the family member. Hospice professionals and volunteers frequently become involved as facilitators and mediators in helping patients and their families to confront realities and meet changing needs in their final times.

Hospice service causes a person to prioritize their values. Hospice services can be uplifting if it leads us to make new friends and learn from patients and their families about how they have lived their lives. Talk about life, past, present, and future, and death, if they bring up the topic, can provide insights into family resilience. My life has been enriched by hearing about the experiences of others, the choices they made, and things they valued, the satisfactions they enjoyed, the challenges they conquered, and the legacies they plan to leave. And how they lived was usually reflected in how they faced death.

We often wait until the end of life to reflect on what is important in life. Then it's too late to do anything about regrets or to spend more time doing what is important to us. Too often we don't stop and take stock of where we are, what we have done, and what we want to accomplish. We are too busy trying to conquer our enemy—time. In the end, time is a friend to those who have valued and used it as the gift that it is.

The purpose of this book is to better understand the role of caregiver and its many dimensions and complexities. The best way to learn about caregiving is to experience its ups and downs and share them so burn-out can be prevented. Since death is the ultimate experience for all of us, it is beneficial to understand care at the end of life better. This book is about what I have learned as a respite volunteer by observing and sharing time with 40 hospice patients and their caregivers at different points in their journeys with time. For some patients, time was an enemy, for others it was a friend, and for still others, time was not important. Our legacy is the story of how we used our time, which is the final gift we share with others.

Families are known to be emotional anchors and to show resilience when problems or crises threaten one of its members. For a family to be told that one of its members has six months or less to live can be devastating. What happens to one family member affects the stability of the family system. Families tend to react to the news of a terminal illness much like they have reacted to other crises. A terminal illness can bring families together or it can tear them apart (Cohen 2008). The reactions of families and their members change as the sick member's illness changes. The needs of the ill person may exceed a family's ability to be sole caregivers. Professional caregivers may be needed in lieu of, or in addition to, family caregivers.

Hospice is not an easy choice for a person and their family to make. Patients and their families may understand that they have a fatal illness but not necessarily that they are dying (Gawande 2014).

The grief process begins when the family learns that a member has a terminal illness. The psychodynamics of the family changes as the primary caregiver is identified; other members of the family may need to change their priorities, roles and responsibilities, and the family and/or its representative decides whether or not they need the additional assistance of professional caregivers. One of the early steps in the grief process is identifying the extent of personal, financial, and other resources needed to help with caretaking (Okun and Nowinski 2011). Families begin to activate their support systems involving extended family, friends, and hospice. Family composition, time demands, and economic constraints will determine the most supportive environment for the patient. A terminal patient may be more comfortable at home under hospice care. An end-of-life prognosis activates different feelings and expectations among family members, especially if the family is geographically dispersed and not closely networked. As a plan is developed to provide caregiving to the family member, the stress of the situation may precipitate feelings of guilt, anger, and family member rivalry. A terminal illness can be a test of family cohesiveness and its long-term stability. The nature of the illness, the amount and type of care needed, the age of the patient, and their values and beliefs all help to shape a personal care plan for the patient.

Sixty-one percent of patients die in hospitals or other acute treatment facilities where extending the length of life is the major objective. Hospice is still a concept and approach that is new to health professionals and laymen. Therefore, patients who enter hospice care do so late in the course of their terminal illnesses (Connor et al. 2007). The U.S. culture still defers to families as the primary caregivers for terminally ill and dying family members. Hospice care can provide a supportive noninvasive environment linked with a philosophy of managing pain and suffering (Carlson et al. 2010; Han et al. 2006; Talley and Crews 2007). Hospice care offers several advantages over traditional hospital-based care for people with terminal illnesses. It can be delivered in a patient's home, allowing death to take place at home, or may optimize the relief of pain, increase patients' satisfaction, and increase cost-effectiveness (Christakis and Escarce 1996).

References

Carlson, M. D. A., Bradley, E. H., Du, Q., & Morrison, R. S. (2010). Geographic access to hospice in the United States. *Journal of Palliative Medicine, 13*(11), 1331–1338.

Christakis, N. A., & Escarce, J. J. (1996). Survival of medicare patients after enrollment in hospice programs. *New England Journal of Medicine, 335*(3), 172–178.

Cohen, R. M. (2008). *Strong at the broken places*. New York: Harper Collins Publishers.

Connor, S. R., Pyenson, B., Fitch, K., & Spence, C. (2007). Comparing hospice and non-hospice patient survival among patients who die within a three-year window. *Journal of Pain and Symptom Management, 33*(3), 238–246.

Gawande, A. (2014). *Being mortal*. New York: Metropolitan Books.

Han, B., Remsburg, R. E., McAuley, M. J., Keay, T. J., & Travis, S. S. (2006). National trends in adult hospice use: 1991–1992 to 1999–2000, *Health Affairs, 25*(3), 792–799.

Kastenbaum, R. (Ed.). (2002). *Macmillan encyclopedia of death and dying* (Vol. 1, 2). New York, USA: Macmillan Reference.

Leary, L. (2012, April 12). No one has to die alone. *Psychology Today*.

Okun, B., & Nowinski, J. (2011). *Saying goodbye: How families can find renewal through loss*. New York: Berkeley Books, Penguin Group (Copyright by Harvard University).

Staudt, C., & Ellens, J. H. (Eds.). (2013). *Our changing journey to the end: Death, dying, and grief in America* (Vol. 1). Santa Barbara, CA: Praeger.

Talley, R. C., & Crews, J. E. (2007). Framing the public health of caregiving. *American Journal of Public Health, 97*(2), 224–228.

Chapter 1
Who are Caregivers?

Abstract Caregivers are present in some form in all societies. An estimated 65.7 million caregivers make up 29 % of the U.S. population providing care to someone who is ill, disabled, or aged. Caregiving is not a simple matter. It is a complex role usually added to other roles a person has in a family. Caregiving can become a long standing and stressful commitment if the family member has a chronic illness. Caregiving is a relationship that is continually changing. Hospice care requires flexible caregiving. In many instances a mix of professional and family caregivers provides care to patients, each contributing their skills, knowledge and support to the patient.

Keywords Becoming a caregiver · Caregivers (defined) · New population of caregivers · Relationships in caregiving

Caregivers are present in some form in all societies. A caregiver is someone who assumes responsibility for the care of an individual who has poor mental health, is physically disabled, or whose health is impaired by sickness or old age. The term "caregiver" may be prefixed with family, spouse, child, parent to distinguish between different care situations and whether the caregiver is a professional or a volunteer. Informal caregivers such as friends, neighbors or family members are unpaid and assist with activities of daily living and tasks in a patient's home. Formal caregivers are paid for providing care at home or in a care setting such as daycare in a residential setting. An estimated 65.7 million caregivers make up 29 % of the U.S. adult population providing care to someone who is ill, disabled, or aged (National Alliance for Caregiving and AARP 2009).

More women than men are caregivers; an estimated 66 % of caregivers are female (Suthers 2006). One-third (34 %) take care of two or more people. The average age of a female caregiver is 48 years (National Alliance for Caregiving and AARP 2009). Men are sharing in caregiving tasks more than in the past, but women still shoulder the major burden of care. Many caregivers of older people are growing older themselves—the average age is 63 years (Marks et al. 2002).

A new population of caregivers to the elderly are children and grandchildren aged 40 and younger. Adults who act as caregivers for both their parents and children are

J.G. Bruhn, *After Diagnosis: Family Caregiving with Hospice Patients*,
SpringerBriefs in Well-Being and Quality of Life Research,
DOI 10.1007/978-3-319-29803-0_1

called the Sandwich Generation. These young adults provide care for their aging parents while supporting their own children (Spillman and Pezzin 2000).

Nearly 80 % of all long-term care is now provided at home by family caregivers to children and adults with serious conditions, including mental illness. Family members who are caregivers provide the foundation for long-term care in the U.S. (Abutaleb 2013; George 1993).

If family caregivers were no longer available, the economic costs to U.S. healthcare and long-term services would increase astronomically. In 2009, about 42.1 million family caregivers in the U.S. provided care to an adult with limitations in daily activities at any given point in time, and about 61.6 million provided care at some time during the year. The estimated economic value of their unpaid contributions was about $450 billion (Family Caregiver Alliance, National Center on Caregiving 2012).

The National Center on Caregiving and AARP (2004) conducted a national survey of 6,139 adults in the U.S. from which 1,247 caregivers were identified in 2003. A profile of caregiving was identified. Caregivers fill multiple roles with the majority (83 %) of caregivers helping family members. The typical caregiver is a 46 year-old woman who has at least some college experience and provides more than 20 h of care each week. Nearly eight in ten care recipients is age 50 or older. More than half (55 %) of care recipients live in their own homes.

Most caregivers say they experience little physical strain (67 %), no emotional stress (44 %) and no financial hardship (77 %). However, caregivers say they provide Level 1 Burden of Care. Analysis showed that the greatest predictors of physical strain are the caregivers own health and whether they feel they had a choice in taking on caretaking responsibilities. Caregivers who report poorer health and those that feel they did not have a choice in taking on the role of caretaker experienced the greatest physical strain. The Level of Burden ranges from Level 1 minimal care to Level 5 maximum care, which contributes to caretaker's physical strain. The greatest influences on caregivers' emotional stress is their Level of Burden, not feeling they had a choice in taking on the role of caregiver, and living in the same household as the person they care for. Almost half of Level 5 caregivers say they need help managing their stress (49 %) and finding time for themselves (53 %).

Wheaton (1990) points out that major life changes and role transitions are often treated as stressors that create a generalized demand for adjustment by an individual. However, transitions have been shown to produce a wide range of effects. Rather than assume that life transitions are inherently stressful, it is useful to determine the social circumstances surrounding "role changes" that influence whether or not a role change or transition is stressful or not. The potential for the impact of a life transition to be stressful is determined by the individual's accumulated experience in the role that is altered by the transition—what can be termed the "role history" prior to the event.

Becoming a Caregiver

Most family caregivers are motivated to assume this role out of love and devotion for the care recipient (Sheehy 2011). But becoming a caregiver is not a simple matter. Caregiving is a complex role usually added to the other roles a person has in a family, such as the role of breadwinner, parent or husband. Caregiving can become a long standing and stressful commitment if the family member has a chronic illness.

Sometimes the caregiver role is assumed somewhat reluctantly if there are no other living relatives who agree to take on this role, especially when the family member's condition worsens and caregiving becomes more demanding.

The caregiver role grows larger in scope and responsibility as the patient's illness changes, especially as the patient becomes more dependent on others for help in performing the tasks of daily life. More people to assist in caregiving will be needed for longer periods of time. Options for help within the family may be limited because of job and personal responsibility in their own lives and limited finances may make it impossible to consider a group home or other environment. The caregiver role can be a source of stress (Scott 2014). Table 1.1 offers some questions and issues for persons considering the caregiver role.

Table 1.1 Some questions and issues a family member needs to consider before agreeing to be a caregiver

1. What is the nature of the patient's illness? What are the patient's care needs now and how are these projected to change? Where is the patient currently residing and what are the current sources of support (physical, fiscal, social-emotional) for the patient? What are the patient's and family's expectations regarding the patient's total care including end-of-life care?
2. What are the limitations of the primary caregiver's ability and qualifications in providing care? If, and when, should professional caregivers become involved in the patient's care? Who are secondary caregivers and resources that could be called upon when needed?
3. Create a care plan for the patient and review and update it daily/weekly
4. What are the family's support resources (financial, respite) available to the primary caregiver? How does the caregiver cope with stress and dying patients? The plan should include respite for the caregiver and professional intervention for the caregiver if needed
5. Caregivers should maintain open communication between themselves, the rest of the family and all involved in the patient's care
6. Caregivers should monitor any changes in the family's attitude about end-of-life care regarding resuscitations and pain management
7. List and compare the burdens (costs) versus the rewards (gains) to becoming a caregiver

The role of caregiver can become increasingly burdensome if the person needing care is permanently disabled and dependent upon others. Indeed, if the patient needs constant supervision for safety concerns, caregiving may involve the entire family. The extent of resources needed such as 24-h care may depend upon the degree to which the family member's illness is debilitating. For example, a family member may suffer a stroke which severely limits his mobility and, in addition, he is diagnosed with Parkinson's disease affecting his movements. For safety reasons he cannot be left alone. Despite his wife's availability as his primary caretaker, and the assistance of hospice professionals and volunteers, he is confined to bed. He has become totally dependent on others; as time has gone on he is now fully bedfast. Limited finances have necessitated the need for home care. His common moods are frustration and anger, and the need for more morphine to manage his aggression and pain. Caregiving has required the involvement of his wife, two hospice nurses, two sons and two volunteers.

Caregivers are needed especially at the end of life. They are essential because they provide needed help with activities of daily living, medications, eating, transportation, emotional support and communicating with health care professionals about the patient's condition. Although there are personal rewards involved for the caregiver, serving as a caregiver over a period of time can be stressful, negatively affecting many aspects of the quality of their own lives (McMillan 2005; Bruhn and Rebach 2014).

Caregiving: A Dynamic Relationship

Caregiving is a relationship that is continually changing; caregivers' initial commitments often need modification as the needs of the patient change. Some patients may only need hospice services for a few days, or weeks, or months, while others exceed their medical projected lifetime by several years. Hospice care requires flexible caregiving, yet there are decision points that characterize most situations (see Fig. 1.1).

The process of hospice caregiving begins with the diagnosis of a terminal illness and an acceptance by the patient and their family that a cure is not possible for the patient's illness. Denial may be the first response to this news. Indeed, hope that the condition can be abated or delayed is often a privately held opinion by the patient and their family. Figure 1.1 indicates that a plan and place for care are the first decisions to be made; a caregiver needs to be identified. The patient's condition will greatly influence the total plan of care and the availability of funds will prescribe the options for where the care can be given (home, group home, nursing home, etc.). The place of care may change as the patient's condition and resources change.

Figure 1.1 points out the relationship between professional (formal) and family (informal) caregivers. In many instances a mix of professional and family caregivers provides care to patients, each contributing their skills, knowledge and support to the patient. The grief process is also part of the total patient care plan including family

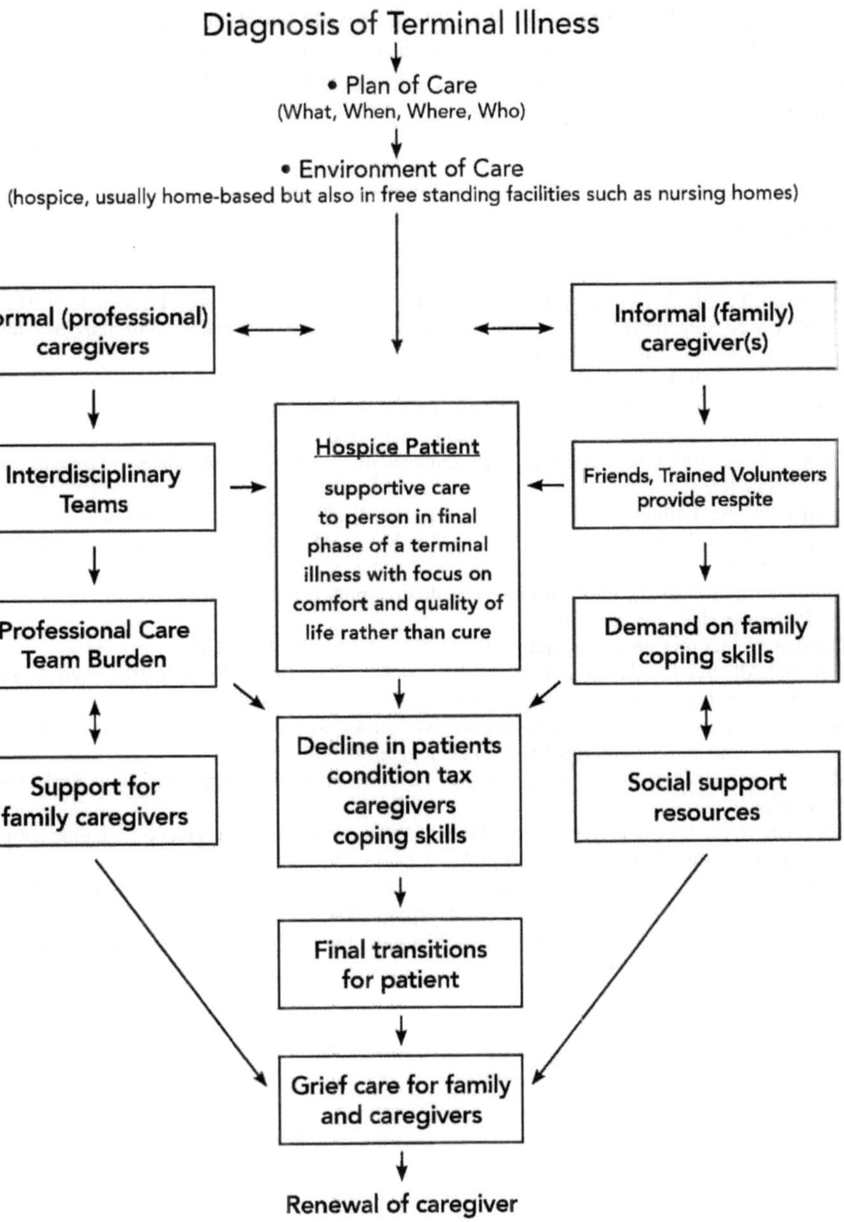

Fig. 1.1 The dynamic relationships and decision points in caregiving to hospice patients

and professional caregivers. Most hospices provide bereavement services following the death of the patient. Services include a variety of support groups, individual counseling, telephone follow-up, and educational materials to help families and caregivers engage in their own renewal.

References

Abutaleb, Y. (2013). Two-fifths of U.S. adults care for sick elderly relatives. Reuters, June 20, 2013. Retrieved September 9, 2014 from http://www.reuters.com/article/2013/06/20/us_usa_health-caregivers-idUSBRE95j03x20130620.

Bruhn, J. G., & Rebach, H. M. (2014). *The sociology of caregiving*. New York: Springer.

Family Caregiver Alliance, National Center on Caregiving (2012). Retrieved September 9, 2014 from https://www.caregiver.org/national-center-caregiving.

George, L. K. (1993). Sociological perspectives on life transitions. *American Sociological Review, 19*, 353–373.

Marks, N. F., Lambert, J. D., & Choi, H. (2002). Transitions to caregiving, gender, and psychological well-being: A prospective U.S. National Study. *Journal of Marriage and Family, 64*, 657–667.

McMillan, S. C. (2005). Interventions to facilitate family caregiving at the end of life. *Journal of Palliative Medicine, 8*(Suppl. 1).

National Center on Caregiving and AARP (2004). Caregiving in the U.S.

National Alliance for Caregiving and AARP (2009). Caregiving in the U.S. Retrieved August 9, 2014 from http://assets.aarp.org/rgcenter/il/caregiving_09_espdf.

Scott, E. (2014). Common causes of caregiver stress. Retrieved January 6, 2014 from http://stress.about.com/od/copingwithcrisis/a/caregiver080507.htm.

Sheehy, G. (2011). *Passages in caregiving: Turning chaos into confidence*. New York: Harper Collins.

Spillman, B. C., & Pezzin, L. E. (2000). Potential and active family caregivers: Changing networks and the Sandwich Generation. *The Milbank Quarterly, 78*(3), 347–374.

Suthers, K. (2006). Women still shouldering the burden: Caregiving in the 21st century. In *National Women's Health Network Newsletter*, May/June 2006.

Wheaton, B. (1990). Life transitions, role histories and mental health. *American Sociological Review, 55*(April), 209–223.

Chapter 2
Time as a Concept in Caregiving

Abstract We have expectations about time and our health. People who have encountered and taken advantage of "the goodness of time" also seem to find peace and comfort in their dying. Seemingly they have few regrets and feel that they have lived successful lives. They used time to benefit themselves and others and have no reason to be regretful or angry about its finality. Examples are offered of how some people "fit living into dying," while others resent the intrusion of dying in their lives. Perceptions of time change when we become ill and are dying.

Keywords Culture and dying · Expectations about time and our health · Perceptions of time · Social support systems

Life is about experiences and relationships. It is what happens when we connect with other people. It is the accumulation of these connections that we call a lifetime in Western cultures. We experience life events and relationships embedded in time. However, not all cultures live with time as we do. Often, when we are immersed in our own culture, it is difficult to understand how people from other cultures perceive our culture, customs, and way of life. In addition, some aspects of our culture are so engrained in our minds and so commonplace to us that we begin to feel that they are universally accepted. One of these cultural variables is how we perceive time. Time has a big effect on interpersonal relationships in a society. In the U.S. for example, life events are embedded in time while the people of Piraha, Brazil, living in the Amazon have no concept of time beyond the present so the concept of future for them doesn't exist. There is no past tense in their language, because everything exists for them in the present. The Piraha's view is in sharp contrast to Americans who often talk of not having enough time and, indeed, may have lingering regrets about not having spent quality time with their families in the past. The Piraha's have no regrets. The core of their culture is simple: "Live here and now." All experience is anchored in the present. Whatever isn't important in the present is quickly forgotten (Levine 1997).

Another South American Amazon people, the Aymara, have had little exposure to outside forces that conflict with their traditional view of time. Aymara culture and

J.G. Bruhn, *After Diagnosis: Family Caregiving with Hospice Patients*,
SpringerBriefs in Well-Being and Quality of Life Research,
DOI 10.1007/978-3-319-29803-0_2

language emphasize the eyewitness point of view, which is literal and straightforward. It's based on the fact that you know where you have been, but you can't know where you are going. So they imagine the past is in front of them where they can see it and the future, which they haven't seen, is behind them.

There are other cultures that can be referred to as "people who live outside of time." The Amondawa tribe, also living in Brazil, does not have a concept of time that can be measured, counted, or talked about in the abstract. Rather they live in a world of serial events, rather than seeing events as being embedded in time. Researchers also found that no one had an age. Instead, they change their names to reflect their stage of life and position within their society, so a little child will give up their name to a newborn sibling and take on a new one. In the U.S. we have so many metaphors for time and its passing that we think of time as "a thing," i.e. "the weekend is almost gone," or "I haven't got the time." We think such statements are objective, but they aren't. We create these metaphors, but the Amondawa don't talk or think in metaphors for time. For the Amondawa they are not time bound or pressured by time. They don't have words or numbers to convey time as an abstract, measurable thing. Time has more to do with experience; and they enjoy freedom from the social expectations that certain life events should occur at certain times or life stages, like the age to marry or begin a family (Palmer 2011).

At the other extreme, the U.S. and many of its Western friends have cultures that are run by time and not surprisingly have the fastest pace. Most people in the U.S. would probably say that they feel rushed. It may be that the ideals and future hopes of American society drive people to be constantly hurried, to reach certain goals by specific times. The epitome of success, luxury, and happiness, often regarded as an illusion, but is a fact, pressured U.S. citizens to constantly do more, earn more, consume more, in order to achieve more. Therefore, for many Americans, free time is less available and, when it is, we often engage in structured competitive activities such as sports, racing etc. Indeed, in the U.S. people are publicly acknowledged and rewarded for being effective managers of time and exceeding expected productivity goals within certain time constraints. As the saying goes, "time is money!" As such, in the U.S., relative chronological boundaries are assigned to life stages or phases, which signal societal expectations regarding marriage, first job, children, stable career and earnings, and retirement. These boundaries, however, can be amended by unexpected forces which delay or permanently change personal and family career goals. Nonetheless, societal expectations regarding time progression along the lifecycle is a force to be acknowledged in a time-driven culture. For example, illness or an accident can delay marriage or having a family and disrupt the "normal" lifecycle progression expected in our society.

In the U.S. and similar time-driven Western cultures the "end of life review" of accomplishments, satisfactions, connections, and wishes often occurs when a person receives a terminal diagnosis. A life review, often used by hospice professionals, can occur spontaneously or it can be structured, it can be painful, but therapeutic, and can culminate in serenity and acceptance of the life one has lived (Jenko et al. 2010).

In Western cultures life reviews are often focused around an individual, but it can take many forms from sharing family histories to healing family conflicts (Remen

1996). Of particular importance is the opportunity to recognize with personal gratitude those persons who have made great contributions to one's life. Time is no longer a constraint to forgiveness and quality time. It is "free" time to examine and appreciate our connections. This freedom is often best experienced in the safe and supportive environment of a self-help group.

It was in a self-help group following her father's death that Betty confessed that she felt so alone although she had lots of relatives. "I feel so disconnected," she said. "Although I come from a big family it was my father who kept us together. He never forgot anyone's birthday; he would pick up the phone to congratulate someone on an accomplishment or write a note to tell someone to have a good day. He was outgoing, always optimistic, happy with a warm smile and a great heart. I didn't do those things. I was quiet and reserved and spent my time developing my career. Now I feel like an orphan. At this stage of my life I don't know how to connect with my own family!"

The group replied, "Connections require commitment. It takes time to connect—you have to decide that it's important and spend time connecting. To enjoy the benefits of connections you have to initiate connections. In order to be loved you have to show love. Too often we realize this too late in life, but there is never a lost moment to connect with others. It is the process of connecting that is important. The benefits will flow from your efforts. Every second of life counts—it is too late to wait until your dying seconds to live your life."

Our perceptions of time change when we become ill and are dying (Neuhaus 2002). We can become disconnected from our environment including family and friends when we no longer have the energy and commitment to maintain our connections and may slip into periods of withdrawal and depression (Cacioppo and Patrick 2008). We need to rely on caregivers who become gatekeepers for deciding with whom we spend our remaining time.

Nearly everyone who is involved in the care of an aging family member experiences grief, although they may not be aware of it. Grieving a loss before it occurs is called "early or anticipatory grief" (Allen 2012). This is a normal process of trying to prepare oneself for the death of a loved one. Anticipatory grief doesn't usually take the place of full-blown grief when the loss occurs. When patients have illnesses over a period of years the outward expression of caregiver grief may appear to be minimal to outsiders, while the survivors' covert reactions to the loss are deeply internalized (Cacioppo and Patrick 2008).

The Limits of Time

Time is paradoxical. Henry Austin Dobson, in 1887, expressed it, "Time goes, you say? Ah no! Alas, time stays, *we* go." For most of us time is viewed as a commodity. We try to organize it, manage it, save it, and remember it. Time is elusive. We seem to either have too much or too little of it, and it moves with speeds that leave us unhappy about both its deficiencies and its excesses. Time seems oblivious to our wants and needs. Time goes on and persists unscathed from our human efforts to control its quantity and quality.

Our personal experience with time also influences our feelings about it. Time is fickle. Sometimes it is our friend, at other times it is our enemy. How we use time influences the outcome of our life experiences, both our accomplishments and our failures. How we evaluate time is closely tied to its meaning in our culture and varies with age, education, gender, and socioeconomic status, and the attitudes of our family, friends, peers and coworkers. How we view time and use it changes as we live our lives. A major lesson we learn about time is that it is a process; it stays and we go! There are multiple dimensions of time, for example there is eternity or timeless time. But our personal time has limits. One of the indicators about the possible quantity and quality of our remaining time is our health. How we use the time and cope with stress, our environment and unplanned events determines the quality and quantity of our lives (Sobel 2004).

Health is a barometer of time. Our health makes us look and feel younger or older than we really are. Older people feel, on average, about 13 years younger than they really are according to a six year study of aging among people between 70 and 104 conducted by the University of Michigan and the Max Planck Institute for Human Development in Berlin (Baltes and Mayer 1990; Baltes and Mayer 2001; Baltes et al. 1993). The aim of the study was to gauge whether the aches and pains of getting older force us to face reality, causing our subjective age to finally catch up with our chronological age. The study found that the very old feel younger than they really are, especially those individuals who were particularly healthy and active. How we feel about age is important because it defines how we act and is associated with our attitudes of hope and well-being (Hirst 2005).

Although we typically think of ourselves as younger than we really are, the study found that most people are not in denial about the aging process. During the course of the six year study, people were asked about their perceptions of age three times. The subjective age wasn't frozen in time, and instead aged with the years. Although the gap typically remained the same, the difference between chronological age and perceived age did begin to narrow as people became less healthy and drew closer to death.

We have expectations about time and our health. Our personalities reflect how we think and feel about our age and health. The effects of aging are both internal and external, nonetheless we pay more attention to the changes we can see. Yet, we have a sixth sense about how time has affected our minds and bodies. We seem "to know" when something is not right with our health. Maybe it's the sudden onset of symptoms, or a comment from a family member or friend about a change in our color, appetite, or energy level that makes us aware of the effects of time on our bodies. While some of us are inclined to deny or dismiss the effects of aging, and delay seeking a medical opinion, others immediately go for an exam. Doctors, after all, intervene to lessen the negative effects of time. They remind us of our accountability for the long-term care of our bodies, minds, and spirits. Not everyone has been a good steward in caring for their health and well-being, therefore, the doctor is not a favorite person on our list of persons to visit.

That was the case of Frank, who had not been to a doctor for several years. Frank had lived 69 years with only minor ailments and no major surgeries. He was overweight and didn't worry about his diet or exercise, but he did have one habit that was beginning to show some physical effects. Frank had inhaled a pack or more of cigarettes a day for the majority of his life, however he had stopped smoking when he retired at age 65. Getting away from the stress of work helped him quit, he said. He had always had what he called a "smoker's cough," experienced shortness of breath, especially with physical activity, a mild degree of wheezing when he breathed, and most recently, tightness in his chest. One Saturday it was the tightness in his chest that he thought was a heart attack that caused him to visit a hospital emergency room. Detailed examination and lung function tests found that Frank had minimized other symptoms such as increased swelling in his ankles, recent weight loss, and lower muscle endurance. He was admitted to the hospital. Frank was diagnosed with severe chronic obstructive pulmonary disease (COPD).

Frank's medical history stated that for many years his symptoms were mild; some he didn't notice or made adjustments in his lifestyle to accommodate them. For the most part Frank had attributed changes, for example, in his decreased mental alertness as signs of aging. Now his symptoms required treatment in a hospital. Frank and his family were told that there was no cure for COPD, that it was progressive and terminal, and would require changes in his lifestyle, such as the use of portable oxygen, not driving a vehicle, and the use of a walker to steady his gait. He would be able to be cared for at home by his family until the recommended treatment for symptoms, that were progressively getting worse, were no longer working. The prognosis of less than one year to live came as a shock to Frank and his family. They were expecting to hear something more hopeful. As they heard the news they knew that all of their lives would be changed. Their sadness and anger prevented them from asking questions. Could the doctor be wrong? Would a second opinion be more hopeful? Was there an experimental treatment that might work or an alternative healer who could talk of hope? How could the news that the person they loved had only a few months to live be real? After all, Frank looked healthy.

Frank and his family drove home in stunned silence. Frank had not felt right for the past year, but had kept his thoughts to himself. He was not prepared for such a short prognosis. He was a person who accepted the fact that, as a male, he might die before his wife, but he never took the time to discuss such an event with his wife. Therefore, Frank had no will, power of attorney, nor had he talked about his end of life wishes, or made any preparations. Now the doctor had explicitly told Frank and his wife to do so.

Frank lapsed into a depression soon after his hospital stay and lost enthusiasm and energy. With the encouragement of his wife they talked openly about what Frank would like to do with his time. He liked the computer, keeping in touch with family and working on the family genealogy. This sharing and networking activity raised his spirits especially as it opened up the opportunity for virtual and face-to-face visits from forgotten or newly-found relatives. Indeed, the entire family environment was transformed from one of gloom to one of optimism and enjoyment, which facilitated the enjoyment of all in planning an end of life celebration for Frank that centered around his wishes.

In addition to facilitating greater family cohesion, Frank's illness also caused family members to become more aware of their diet, weight and daily health habits such as exercise, sleep and stress management. The entire family had become fully involved in Frank's caregiving. To prevent caregiver burnout Frank agreed to enroll in a local hospice that provided at-home care including a nurse who monitored vital signs, medications, and equipment needs, a nurse's aide who helped Frank in his activities of daily living, and a hospice volunteer who became a friend and provided weekly respite for Frank's caregivers. Indeed, hospice provided an additional layer of social and emotional support for the family. Time became less of a burden as the extended social network embraced Frank and helped maximize his quality of life. Frank died peacefully, as the family held his hands and the family dog lay at his feet, just as he had wished.

Time is a measure of the quality of our lives. Time shapes us from birth to death. There is some truth to "being in the right place at the right time." Opportunists and optimists are particularly skilled at sensing the "right" time to intervene to seize the particular benefits from situations and people. They seem to make time work for them in positive ways. Indeed, life's successes are often due to the degree of astuteness a person has in understanding that time never repeats itself in the same way. Success is the accumulation of select moments in time, which, in turn, create other select moments. Time is a process so we can't go back and relive it, or save it. Regrets are missed opportunities in reading time.

On the other hand, people who have encountered and taken advantage of "the goodness of time" also seem to find peace and comfort in their dying (Buchwald 2006). Seemingly they have few regrets and feel they have lived successful lives. They used time to benefit themselves and others and have no reason to be regretful or angry about its finality.

Fitting Living into Dying

Mary's motorized wheelchair conveyed her strong feelings about being independent and active. At age 97 she lived in her own apartment in an assisted living facility. Her weekly schedule of talking with family, visitors, bridge, entertainment events, and spiritual time, was a denial that congestive heart failure was applicable to her. She did acquiesce to the part-time assistance of a helper who prepared meals and arranged transportation to medical appointments, but insisted in being in charge of her life. After a recent hospitalization her family was unsuccessful in getting her to talk about her wishes for the end of her life. Whatever preparations she had made she kept to herself.

Her bed seemed insignificant in the room where she spent most of the day where a desk piled high with papers, correspondence, and pending fiscal matters was readily accessible to her. The bedroom walls were covered with pictures of family members—her late husband, sons and their families, significant events of the grandchildren, including pets, all conveying loving memories, smiles of happiness, and gratitude for her support and contributions to their lives. In between the pictures were small plaques of religious quotes and sayings conveying hope and the importance of a positive attitude in life.

She looked forward to each new day. It was part of each day's routine that she get connected with her portable oxygen, put in her hearing aides, find her glasses, put on make-up and get settled in her wheelchair before she started a conversation—which was always a question about how the other person was doing. She didn't wear a watch and there were no clocks within sight to make time important. Her stamina determined the frequency and duration for visits. Pain, fatigue or her disease were never brought up as topics for conversation.

Mary fit living into her dying. The progressive effect of age, rather than illness, was a challenge to living a full life. She never talked about death, her fears (if any) or beliefs; she lived as if life was a seamless progression of events to be shared and remembered. So it was, she died alone during her sleep, in her bedroom, with her artifacts of a life fully lived.

The diagnosis of a chronic, progressive disease brings out the pessimism or optimism in people. Pessimists seem to give into their disease concluding that their future plans are limited and there is little hope since there is no cure for their disease. Optimists, on the other hand, conclude that there is always hope and each moment should be lived as if it were the last. Indeed, some believe that retaining a zest for life, and being grateful for their life so far, are strong enough to make plans; they may realize some of their dreams and goals. A progressive, chronic disease need not be a death sentence. Diseases, like the individuals who have them, have different attributes that make them unique in their effects and consequences. We have all seen the variability of the progression of chronic diseases; likewise we have all seen patients surrender to their disease, while others become motivated to fight even more.

Much of our attitude toward disease is influenced by our social support system. If we face our illness alone, we feel its effects more keenly—when there are not others who can provide encouragement and hope. If we have a strong support system, which includes visitors, cards, and family taking the patient out for a visit to a park, a ball game, or a restaurant, we feel more connected and hopeful. Hospice personnel, especially volunteers, can be a reliable source of friendship and support (Sheehy 2010).

Illness affects our perceptions of time and what to expect from it, yet we all have the same amount of it. The use of time is very personal, some people feel chronically robbed of time, while others have time on their hands. Our views about time and how we use it change as we age and our lives fill up with new responsibilities and demands. We still have the same amount, we merely value time differently and portion it out to meet new and changing priorities. Therefore, a terminal illness can change the length of a life, it need not change our attitudes towards life or how we live it. It is possible to fit living into dying.

And living, despite the limitations of his various illnesses, was what Bob was determined to do. He was not sure what being a newly admitted hospice patient was all about; it was his new doctor and wife who convinced him that hospice would provide a wider range of services than where he had been enrolled and unhappy. He especially liked the option for a volunteer to provide respite for his wife and he could continue to live at home. Several falls precipitated a concern about Bob's safety; he needed a walker to support his slight frame and unsteady gait.

In his mid-seventies, Bob had a varied career as a business owner after his service in the Air Force. He enjoyed telling stories about WWII, especially the time he met and married his wife. His long oxygen line permitted him to retrieve several models of various airplanes which have a prominent place in his bedroom. He cups his right ear and leans forward to engage in a conversation while telling the listener he can't read due to macular degeneration. Bob is also a lung cancer survivor; he says he smoked as much as five packages of cigarettes a day for most of his life. He now has Chronic Obstructive Pulmonary Disease, but sneaks a cigarette on the patio when his wife is out running errands.

Bob's pleasures in life are travelling, gambling, and good restaurants. He and his wife have enjoyed many vacations to Europe. Visits to casinos are feasible for a few hours of blackjack a few times a month as long as his stamina holds out, which is determined by whether he is winning or not. And Bob and his wife also enjoy weekly visits to restaurants. The closeness of the family is evident in the numerous pictures of their children and grandchildren that are grouped along the walls of their living and family rooms.

Bob's dry sense of humor helps him keep his emotional balance. He humors his wife who he worries about because she is so protective and caring of him. Bob says his wife needs the respite and can get out of the house to be with her friends.

References

Allen, J. (2012). *The Long Road: An Article on Anticipatory Grief.* Retrieved November 9, 2014, from http://www.google.com/search7client=safari&ris=en&g=Allen+J+2012The+Long+Road&le=UTF.UTF-&&oe=UTF-8.

Baltes, P. B., & Baltes, M. M. (Eds.). (1990). *Successful aging: Perspectives from the behavioral sciences*. Cambridge: Cambridge University Press.

Baltes, P. B., & Mayer, K. U. (Eds.). (2001). *The Berlin aging study: Aging from 70 to 100* (2nd ed.). New York: Cambridge University Press.

Baltes, P. B., Mayer, K. U., Helmchen, H., & Steinhagen-Thiessen, E. (1993). The Berlin Aging Study (BASE): overview and design. *Ageing and Society, 13*, 483–515.

Buchwald, A. (2006). *Too soon to say goodbye*. New York: Random House.

Cacioppo, J. T., & Patrick, W. (2008). *Loneliness*. New York: W. W. Norton & Co.

Hirst, M. (2005). Carer distress: A prospective, population-based study. *Social Science in Medicine, 61*, 697–708.

Jenko, M., Gonzalez, L., & Alley, P. (2010). Life review in critical care: Possibilities at the end of life. *Critical Care Nurse, 30*(1), 17–27.

Levine, R. A. (1997). *A geography of time*. New York: Basic Books.

Neuhaus, R. J. (2002). *As I lay dying*. New York: Basic Books.

Palmer J. (2011). Amondawa Tribe Lacks Abstract Idea of Time. BBC News. May 29, 2011.

Remen, R. N. (1996). *Kitchen table wisdom: Stories that heal*. New York: Berkeley Publishing Group.
Sheehy, G. (2010). *Passages in caregiving: Turning chaos into confidence*. New York: Harper Collins.
Sobel, R. K. (2004). The time before dying. *U.S. News and World Report, 19*, 2004.

Chapter 3
The Emotional Roller Coaster of Caregiving

Abstract Caregiving is a journey itself. It is not surprising that some caregivers physically and emotionally deplete themselves in giving care to a patient and become sick or die prematurely. The type of illness and a patient's personality along with the composition of the family, its ethnicity and culture all interact to create an emotional roller coaster. The most common emotions that illness produces in patients and families are anxiety, depression, fear, and hopelessness. The deepest feelings about caregiving, which are often unspoken, especially among family, are related to finances. The financial burden of caregiving is the most changeable, inflatable, and unplanned aspect of long-term care.

Keywords Caregiver emotions · Cumulative effects of chronic disease · Family communication · Limits of family caregiving

It is common for a patient's caregiver and family members to experience the emotional roller coaster ride of a patient's chronic illness. Seeing the cumulative effects of a progressive disease on a loved one can be so emotionally draining that the caregiver also becomes victimized by the disease. Patients, on the other hand, may not be aware of their emotional ups and downs because they have incorporated the disease and its effects into their personalities. The ill person's disease, therefore, becomes their identity.

Don's wife and two daughters had just settled into their new spacious home when they began to notice subtle changes in Don's behavior. He seemed to be increasingly anxious and frustrated, and experienced memory problems. This was a marked change from his behavior as CEO of a large corporation, which required predictability and planning. Indeed, Don frequently became argumentative and abusive toward family members leading to a visit to the family physician. A neurology consult affirmed the early stages of Parkinson's dementia. The prognosis was devastating to the family who were looking forward to early retirement, and a life of travel and hiking. Perhaps the most damaging effect of the diagnosis was how daily family activities were shaped by Don's mood and behavior on a given day. The family had to arrange their schedules around Don's

J.G. Bruhn, *After Diagnosis: Family Caregiving with Hospice Patients*,
SpringerBriefs in Well-Being and Quality of Life Research,
DOI 10.1007/978-3-319-29803-0_3

changing needs. The family became a prisoner to Don's disease, and to further complicate communication within the family, Don was often unaware of his behavior and its effects on others. Medication controlled Don's symptoms to some degree, but the underlying disease was progressive.

Over the course of the year following the initial diagnosis, Don became more agitated, continuously moving from room to room with his walker as he heard noises and communicated with unseen others in the house. Because of the high risk of falling, someone had to be with Don constantly as he moved quickly. Medication had only mediating effects. The psychological impact of seeing Don deteriorate and the tensions in addressing his continual needs, left his wife and daughters emotionally fragile. Sometimes they were the targets of Don's hurtful comments, his uncooperativeness, and his attempts to leave them. This often caused family members to shout at one another and to blame one another for Don's neglect and decline. The family became fractured. Don's wife sought counseling, a daughter left home; they saw and talked to each other less often. Hospice provided needed daytime respite care from volunteers that was supplemented by 24-h nursing care. Eventually Don had to be placed in a total care facility. The family's feelings of guilt about having to move Don to a facility increased the family's fragility. Don settled into his new living quarters and, while he did not understand why he was no longer at home, he looked forward to frequent family visits (Wilbur 1988).

Caregiving is a journey itself. It is not surprising that some caregivers physically and emotionally deplete themselves in giving care to a patient and become sick or die prematurely. Compassion often creates everyday heroes, however, caregiving has its limits. Most illnesses create a cycle of emotions for patients and families that parallel the course of the disease. The type of illness and a patient's personality along with the composition of the family, its ethnicity and the culture in which it is embedded all interact to create an emotional roller coaster. Since families and patients experience illness differently there is no prototype of emotions that apply to all families or patients.

Perhaps the most common emotions that illness produces in patients and families are anxiety, depression, fear, and hopelessness. These are common emotions because they relate to the uncertainty and unpredictability of illness, especially chronic illnesses. Most patients adapt to their illness more readily when the family is cohesive and supportive. Like a rubber band emotions can be retracted and expanded; the give and take of the patient and their family is key to the successful long term care of chronic conditions (Brown et al. 2003).

The deepest feelings about caregiving, which are often unspoken, especially among family, are related to finances. If the patient is older it is likely insurance coverage for long-term care is inadequate or non-existent. This means, dependent upon the patient's needs and the family's willingness to supplement or pay fully for health care, the patient may need to be cared for in their home instead of a facility or be moved to a lower cost facility as finances dwindle. It is not uncommon that group homes, for example, can cost $5,000 or more a month. Family members may not all be able or willing to help financially which can cause family friction and estrangement among members. Some family members may be concerned about their share of inheritance being devoted to the cost of extended care for a dying parent. Financial worries feed into the overall emotional drain of long-term caregiving.

Indeed, the financial burden of caregiving is the most changeable, inflatable, and unplanned aspect of long-term care. Yet, as people live longer with chronic conditions and the cost of health care increases, the majority of Americans will be confronted by cost dilemmas several times within a family generation.

References

Brown, S. L., Nesse, R. M., Vinokur, A. D., & Smith, D. M. (2003). Providing social support may be more beneficial than receiving it: Results from a prospective study of mortality. *Psychological Science, 14*(4), 320–327.

Wilbur, K. (1988). On being a support person. *The Journal of Transpersonal Psychology, 20*(2), 141–158.

Chapter 4
Dying Is a Team Effort

Abstract Death is the end of a series of transitions. The time of dying is highly individualistic. Not all people have the opportunity or wish to plan their own funerals or celebration of life services. Whatever the circumstances or personal desires regarding the dying process, professional caregivers usually present grievers with choices regarding how their family member dies. Hospice provides an 11th hour companion to be with the patient to provide respite for family, or to be a companion when family cannot be physically present with the patient. Often older people may be in a hospital, nursing or group home and in the absence of family, they end up dying alone.

Keywords Celebration of life · Dying with hospice · Patient wishes in dying · Planning in dying

Bedridden and dying from pulmonary fibrosis, 67 year old Tom had a vision of his funeral and he was determined to plan the event in every detail. He shocked many of his lifelong friends when they received his phone call to be a pallbearer or to speak at his funeral. He selected the music, who would sing and who would play the piano. With the assistance of his parish priest he selected biblical quotations and the theme of the homily. He selected charities to receive the money that ordinarily would be spent on flowers. He convinced his wife of her need to develop the bulletin for the service, which had a photo of Tom on its cover. A table of photos of family members and friends taken during happier times, would greet the guests at the entrance to the church. All church members were to be invited.

Tom had all necessary papers regarding his will, power of attorney and the allocation of his possessions finalized so no details except their implementation burdened any family member. During the weeks of the planning for his funeral Tom became energized and chuckled at the memories he reawakened. He relished "being in charge" and coordinating the many players who reported on their assigned part in his funeral plan. Even the family dog knew when to jump on the bed and become a participant.

J.G. Bruhn, *After Diagnosis: Family Caregiving with Hospice Patients*,
SpringerBriefs in Well-Being and Quality of Life Research,
DOI 10.1007/978-3-319-29803-0_4

Tom became sicker and needed greater amounts of medication for his pain, and the harpist from hospice came to play some of his favorite pieces. The dog spent more time lying at the foot of the bed. Tom died quietly with members of his funeral planning team circling the bed while the priest blessed him.

Not all people have the opportunity or wish to plan their own funerals. Funerals, memorial services or celebrations of life are usually tailored to the personality of the deceased and their wishes. It is often considered an act of love if relatives would address the topic, even if painful, while the patient is conscious and of a relatively clear mind. Indeed celebrations of life are often considered a positive way to characterize the legacy desired by the deceased.

A 2007 Harris poll showed that 55 % of Americans die without a will. For whatever personal reasons some people do not want to plan for their death and ease decision-making among their family members. For others, death is the final transition in the lifecycle and a time to involve others in emotionally sharing the dying person's legacies. Many people are grateful for the demonstration of care and support of others as they make this final transition. Some people are alone because their families have preceded them in death or they have chosen a single lifestyle. Whatever the circumstances of personal desires regarding the dying process, professional caregivers usually present grievers with choices regarding how their family member dies. Hospice, for example, may provide an 11th hour companion to be with the patient to provide respite for family or be a companion when family cannot be physically present with the patient. Often older people who may be in a hospital, nursing home or group home may be the sole living family member and therefore end up dying alone (Schulz and Beach 1999).

Death is the end of a series of life transitions (Kubler-Ross 1969). While it is a sad time due to the loss of a loved one, too often death is viewed negatively and fearfully. In some people's view it seems death is a failure, yet, if lived fully, a life lived should be celebrated. It can be a time to recall good memories, and contributions left behind.

Death may be sudden or prolonged; in the later instance there is the luxury of added time to plan a celebration of life with the possible participation of the dying person themselves. We all die whether we plan for it or not. Planning for death gives us the opportunity to share our hopes. The time of dying is highly individualistic in its meaning even when we share it, but in verbal sharing we leave a more personal legacy.

References

Kubler-Ross, E. (1969). *On Death and Dying*. New York: Touchstone.

Schulz, R., & Beach, S. R. (1999). Caregiving as a risk factor for mortality: The Caregiver Health Effects Study. *Journal of the American Medical Association, 282*(23), 2215–2219.

Chapter 5
Spirit: The Timekeeper

Abstract The will to live is considered to be one of the basic drives in man; some health professionals believe that it plays an important role in one's chances for survival and increased longevity. In essence spirit gives life to our personhood. Some health professionals believe that spirit is important in maintaining good health and in coping with illness. Spirit can be supported and strengthened outside of a person, but the essence of spirit cannot be rehabilitated or replaced since it is the basis of our personhood. Spirit is our reason for living. It is our timekeeper.

Keywords Life satisfaction · Process of dying · Time as a gift · Spirit

Spirit is the life-giving and unifying part of the mind-body dyad that gives purpose and direction to our lives. Spirit is with us at birth and leaves us at death. Spirit is sometimes considered to be analogous to soul or the will to live. The will to live is considered to be one of the basic drives in man; some health professionals believe that it plays an important role in one's chances for survival and increased longevity.

Spirit helps to shape personality; it conveys who we are and why we are here. High-spirited people tend to be more energetic, enthusiastic and courageous than would be expected in most people. Spirit is conveyed in our interpersonal relationships with others and is intrinsic to our beliefs and desires; high-spirited people convey a sense of coherency or "having it together." In essence, spirit gives life to our personhood. Some physicians and psychologists believe that spirit is essential in maintaining good health and in coping with illness; it is the "bounce-back" factor that helps people recover from adversity.

Alice had spirit. Staff and other patients at the nursing home frequently came to her room where they found a smile, were given an optimistic greeting and an invitation to sit down in the single over-stuffed chair. The nearby chest of drawers was covered with cards, family photos, stuffed animals and nick-knacks—each having a story to tell. And Alice was a storyteller. Storytelling could keep her from selectively eating her institutional meal.

For the most part Alice was wheelchair bound, but she took both a morning and afternoon tour of her unit with the assistance of a walker and aide to keep connected

J.G. Bruhn, *After Diagnosis: Family Caregiving with Hospice Patients*,
SpringerBriefs in Well-Being and Quality of Life Research,
DOI 10.1007/978-3-319-29803-0_5

with her network of friends and informed of the latest personnel changes. Alice didn't need the daily paper, magazine or television for her information; she preferred face-to-face interaction. She had daily visits from her daughter and son-in-law who frequently took her out to her favorite restaurant.

At age 88 Alice had already experienced loss. Her husband died previously and an aging sister lived independently in her home in another state; they had stayed connected for the last few years by phone. Alice had moved to be near her only child, a daughter, who cared for her at home until recently when they agreed that Alice needed nursing and hospice care. Despite Alice's general debility, her mind was sharp, her optimism remained strong, and her spirit was unbreakable. One day that all changed. Alice was found depressed and crying silently as she slumped in her wheelchair. Her daughter had just been diagnosed with malignant stomach cancer. Alice had said, "a mother is not supposed to live to attend her daughter's funeral." The disease progressed rapidly and Alice's daughter joined her mother as a hospice patient. The hospice volunteer arranged transportation for Alice to see her daughter at home before the daughter's death. They spent an entire day together.

Alice lost some of her vitality after her daughter's death; she requested hospice care. Alice's son-in-law did his best to fill the void his wife left—he visited Alice frequently, brought her meals, and provided emotional support. But in Alice's view, there was nothing to live for anymore—she seemed to give up. She slept more, ate less, and the stoop in her back became more pronounced as she made her daily tours around the unit. Her son-in-law remarried. It was within a few months of her daughter's death that Alice died peacefully in her sleep. Alice had a strong religious faith and hope that sustained her, but as she said, "I am ready to go anytime."

Spirit can be supported and strengthened by resources outside a person, but the essence of spirit cannot be rehabilitated or replaced, as it is the basis of our personhood. Spirit is our reason for living. It is our timekeeper. We cannot give someone more time. What is essential is that we respect and facilitate the quality of time each person has as they move along life's transitions.

The time at which the different stages of life occur and the occurrence of life events differ among cultures. For example, in some cultures adolescence is very short and the expectations of adulthood come more quickly than in other cultures. This means that events such as the birth of a child and marriage may come at an early stage of life, e.g. adolescence. Likewise, in countries with a low life expectancy, death may occur commonly in the 40s or 50s while in countries with high life expectancy there are many more centenarians. Culture influences peoples' expectations regarding life transitions and their passage. Cultures vary also in how much personal control they can exert during the various transition periods of one's life. For example, Buddhism teaches how to consciously control the processes of dying, death, and rebirth. In general, in American society, while there are differences in religious beliefs about death, it is viewed as the final transition in one's earthly life-cycle. Irrespective of one's belief in an afterlife, in the U.S. death is culturally considered a negative experience in that it is a loss, albeit for some, temporary. The process of dying can vary enormously from a prolonged, painful one to a sudden, unexpected one. There is much variation in dying because it is highly individualistic with uncertainties tied to the culture, religion, and personality of the dying person. It is difficult, therefore, to generalize observations from dying experiences. Even people who have died and been resuscitated report different experiences.

Death is often the final phase of an illness or follows the complications of an accident. In the former instance death may be expected and considered timely while in the latter case it occurs unexpectedly and is considered untimely. Nonetheless, death in the U.S. is usually considered a shock. Death is a shock even when it occurs among hospice patients. We seem to be emotionally unprepared for it even when we intellectually expect it. No one is guaranteed a "full life," or a long one, however these may be defined. How one spends his/her time, therefore, is the key to judging its completeness, which should be a commentary and not a debate (Byock 1997, 2012).

Bill was a large man and a formidable athlete in his time. He had lived an active, vigorous life and traveled the globe in his work. At age 91, however, loss of strength in his legs confined him to a wheelchair. His family was young and active yet they couldn't care for him so he was transferred to a group home. He kept to himself in his room except at mealtime when he interacted minimally at the kitchen table with the other four residents. A hospice team visited him weekly. He mentioned that he was due to have his 91st birthday and had never had a birthday party. Much to his shock and delight on his birthday, cards, balloons, a birthday cake and music greeted him at the dining table. He read and re-read his cards. A few days later he developed trouble swallowing and was admitted to the hospital where he developed complications and died.

Bill was a person of few words, a keen sense of humor, sharp insight, and a clear mind. He revealed his life story as a photographer of international note, but kept no photos of his life. He never spoke of death, or dying, or regrets, only how kind time had been to him and his family.

Dying More Than Once

Two real life stories about resuscitation following death offer the range of perspectives people have about getting "extra time" or "a second chance at life." A professor of medicine collapsed and fell unconscious during a lecture he was giving to a class of medical students. The students revived him. The professor used to joke about how important it was to be in the right place when one dies. He lived many years to teach other classes of medical students. At the opposite extreme was a patient with severe cardiac problems who stopped breathing while in the hospital. A Code Blue team successfully resuscitated the patient only to meet his fury when the doctors told him he had been revived. He said, "I died legitimately and you brought me back to life"!

Time has a different value for each of us depending on our age, our general health, our quality of life, our resources, the extent to which we have met our life goals, experienced our dreams, and our remaining hopes and aspirations (Callanan and Kelley 1992). And then there are our personalities; how much fight and hardiness we have left in us, or what is sometimes called “the will to live.” There are people who do not want interventions to extend their life, while others don’t want to give in or give up. Either extreme has its problems; some people lose their zest for life and their ability to cope with it. Sometimes these people are the sole survivors in their families and they are lonely, tired and have lost a positive meaning for living. Sometimes people want repeated interventions in order to live because of their love for life, its remaining challenges, and a strong family support system. Most caregivers will be able to assess their patient’s “spirit for living” after a few days or weeks of caregiving.

Jerry’s large frame filled the recliner where he spent almost every day during the past year monitored by his two large dogs, napping, watching TV, and visiting with friends. Retired from the military he had many stories to tell about his past and enjoyed the attention of having someone listen to him. His mild dementia enabled him to retell certain parts of some stories for emphasis. His wife worked and relied on hospice caregivers to care for him. His vision and hearing were poor so whoever was present needed to sit close to him. The walls in his corner of the family room were covered with diplomas, certificates of praise, medals in framed boxes, and a large stack of scrapbooks. He had written his life story as a book, his wife typed it, and he self-published it. Jerry never talked about dying, yet his diabetes, cardiac and lung diseases, and decreased mobility emphasized his dependence on others and pointed to a steady decline. Weekly visits by clergy from the church where he was a charter member affirmed his unwavering beliefs about a better life after death. But for the present Jerry monitored the daily activities of a charity he organized which distributed toys to the less fortunate at Christmas. The continuing success of the charity was his legacy.

The DNR (Do Not Resuscitate) order taped on the refrigerator made it clear that Jerry was firm about dying only once. He believed that he had lived a full and satisfying life and he did not want to be resuscitated and possibly be a greater caregiving burden to his wife and family. End of life issues were freely discussed, decisions were made, and never revisited or regretted. Jerry said, “Every moment should be lived with as much joy as possible, and every day should be one of satisfactions, beyond that it’s in God’s hands.”

Time: The Great Equalizer

To be born and to die are not decisions we make. We are accountable to others, and ourselves however, for how we used our time between birth and death. As we reflect on our lives there are several key principles we learn about time, specifically our time.

Time is a process that is influenced by many intrinsic and extrinsic factors. Moments occur sequentially. We can’t relive time or save it. We can only live for the moment. Our actions or inactions at a given moment may influence subsequent actions or inactions so that moments become cumulative in their effects. Our use of time is affected by life events both those in and outside of our control. As we periodically reflect on our use of time we make changes in our goals, expectations, and hopes. As we age we increasingly realize that time is a gift that is about living. We can only experience time as it happens—its speed, its quality and its opportunities. We learn that we are users, not creators of time.

How we have used our collective time is often the basis for reflecting upon the degree of satisfaction and meaningfulness we feel we have achieved in our lives. No one escapes the regrets, hurts, or dissatisfactions in life or its pleasurable experiences and memories. Yet, a balanced perspective of a life of satisfaction is often put to a test when a person receives the news of a terminal diagnosis, especially if it is chronic, painful, and requires extensive caregiving. Time often carries caveats beyond the normal expected effects of aging and its disabilities. A terminal illness and its time compression undoubtedly have profound social, emotional, physical, and financial effects on a person and their family. On the other hand, the use of time is uniquely individualistic and a terminal diagnosis may move a family toward greater cohesion in the care of the patient. For some patients a terminal diagnosis creates embitterment and anger such that offers of assistance are rejected by the patient resulting in their greater suffering. The goal of hospice is to help patients make friends with time and lessen pain and suffering.

Time may not always heal, but time changes us. It changes our perspective, our feelings, our honesty. It is our changed feelings that make pain more painless. Caregivers and volunteers give time as a gift; it has value for them, the patient and the patient's family.

End times cause us to respect and value relationships. Too often hurts are hidden, regrets are suppressed, negative emotions are denied in the presence of the dying only to be faced later in a grief self-help group. Sometimes we are too late in expressing our love and gratitude to the dying if we find them unconscious and unresponsive. Therefore, the best practice is to go to bed each night with a forgiving heart and a commitment to make "quality time" for those we value as a high priority (Vitaliano et al. 2003).

References

Byock, I. (1997). *Dying well*. New York: Riverhead Books.
Byock, I. (2012). *The best care possible*. New York: Avery.
Callanan, M., & Kelley, P. (1992). *Final gifts*. New York: Bantam Books.
Vitaliano, P. P., Zhang, J., & Scanlan, J. M. (2003). Is caregiving hazardous to one's physical health? A meta-analysis. *Psychological Bulletin, 129*(6), 946–972.

Chapter 6
Holding on and Giving Up

Abstract In Western culture "holding on" is usually thought of as showing strength. It has been said that "all of the art of living lies in the mingling of letting go and holding on." Some people think that it's "holding on" that makes one strong, but sometimes it's "letting go." Letting go doesn't mean that you are giving up but rather accepting that there are things we cannot change. "Giving up" on the other hand, means the suspension of the will to live or there is no longer an attempt made to deal with life's challenges or to look ahead. Not all deaths have equal importance to the family system, but all families need to grieve to cope with loss.

Keywords Family as a system · Family repertoire of social support · Grieving · Holding on

Medicare guidelines state that to be eligible for a hospice benefit, patients must be in their last six months of life. More recently Medicare has changed its rules for admission to hospice to make the process more flexible and to recognize that it is difficult to predict how long a patient will live. Therefore, it is not surprising that patients are referred for hospice care late in the progression of their illness. The average length of stay is less than one month. Doctors may not always recognize when patients need hospice care (Kleinman 2008). There is some reluctance on the part of patients and their families to decide the time for hospice care. Such a decision may be considered by the patient as "giving up" since they would no longer receive palliative chemotherapy, radiation therapy, or some of the more expensive medications. Ironically, it is not unusual for some patients admitted to hospice to feel better and become more functional as they receive more social support, at least in the short term. Some patients and physicians are not aware that patients who were admitted to hospice can be discharged if they live beyond hospice guidelines, and then readmitted when they begin to decline again. This process is, however, unsettling for patients and their families, since it often involves geographical relocation, equipment and treatment changes, and social disconnections with caregivers. There is some research that found that one-third of the patients who were discharged from a hospice died within six months (Span 2014).

J.G. Bruhn, *After Diagnosis: Family Caregiving with Hospice Patients*,
SpringerBriefs in Well-Being and Quality of Life Research,
DOI 10.1007/978-3-319-29803-0_6

The processes of "holding on," "letting go," and "giving up" are often thought, but not verbally expressed in the presence of the dying. In our culture "holding on" is usually thought of as showing strength. This is usually the thought of a family member who wants the dying person to show strength by not giving into a disease, but it often has more to do with unresolved issues the survivor has that they haven't addressed with the dying person or with the survivor's ambivalence about assuming control of the dying person's estate or responsibilities. "Holding on" gets increasingly difficult to do, and it is an unrealistic expectation of a dying person who does not have control of his life. Very often a patient can choose the day of death. Statistics suggest that people can postpone death until after a holiday, or birthday, or anniversary. They often can will themselves to live for a time that has great significance for them. As one family said of their dying spouse, "We kept telling him, the holidays are over. It's ok., you can let go now."

Psychologist Havelock Ellis said, "All the art of living lies in the mingling of letting go and holding on." Some people think that it's "holding on" that makes one strong, but sometimes it's "letting go." Letting go doesn't mean you are giving up, but rather accepting that there are things we cannot change. "Giving up," on the other hand, means the suspension of the will to live or there is no longer an attempt made to deal with life's challenges or to look ahead. Giving up often shows a lack of courage.

What is important for hospice patients and their families is to use the time in hospice to openly and frankly discuss the patient's issues, and those of their survivors, while they are still competent and conscious.

The Family—A Healing System

A death, irrespective of how expected or how peaceful, leaves wounded survivors. The family is a system of relationships and every family member reacts to the death of a family member somewhat differently, depending upon their relationship with the deceased member. The family is an interactive unit, a system of relationships. The roles the deceased played are key in understanding the impact of the death the member has on the functioning of the entire family. A death can enhance family cohesion and resilience or create new tensions or fractures. Indeed, the absence of a family member through death can cause some family members to revive conflicts or begin new ones. Members can triangulate or pair off rather than work together as a unit. The existing leader or a new one in the family needs to emerge to arbitrate and resolve conflict. Death will usually activate the coping devices individuals and families used in dealing with previous family crises. Sometimes healing can occur through the efforts of the family collectively, without the assistance of a professional outside the family. Nonetheless, most mental health experts will agree that adaptation to a death depends upon the degree of resilience of a family and its members, and their collective will to strengthen and sustain family bonds (Poulin et al. 2010).

A family's behavior at the death of a member can only be understood as a part of its history. This involves understanding a family's coping strategies as a system in response to past stressors. Patterns of adaptation of families and individual members develop over time and are transmitted across family generations. How a family organized itself around previous crises is a strong predictor about how they will behave in other crises. Unexpected death, such as that of a child, often taxes the coping responses of a family especially if the family is currently dealing with additional crises. This is why support systems are so important in providing some balance and respite in coping with long term crises such as a prolonged death.

It is important to know a family's repertoire of social support, its availability, and the family's ability to use them. No family is strong or healthy enough to cope with the event of death by itself. Every family has hidden risks, which need to be revealed and used preventively so there are no later surprises.

The goal of bringing about healing to a grieving family is to help it restore itself to as natural a rhythm as possible. Duties and responsibilities in a family can be reallocated, but people who performed them previously are not replaceable—every person performs their roles uniquely. Therefore, it is important to know, from a systems point of view, the place of the family lifecycle and stage of development of all family members. Each family member's ability to adapt and the rates at which he/she does is directly related to each individual's own development and role(s) in the family.

Many family's adjustment difficulties from death originate in the lack of openness in the system, that is, the ability of each family member to communicate their feelings to others and to act on them. Families that are able to communicate, share information and options, and use external support networks such as friends, counseling, and self-help groups, especially when grief is prolonged and intense, are less likely to become dysfunctional than families that are less open and connected with others.

Every family has its own family "fabric"—texture, style, and ability to withstand death and similar stresses. Interventions can be helpful to families with unresolved mourning. The resources of hospice are especially helpful in dealing with appropriate feelings and tasks of death and dying and moving on with their lives.

John was a small man with a big spirit, lots of energy, a sharp mind, devilish eyes, and a no-nonsense attitude. He had a list of things medically wrong with him, but it was only recently when he was diagnosed with congestive heart failure and had to carry portable oxygen that he gave into receiving hospice care at home. He fought hard when he gave up his cane for a walker. He loved people and people loved to visit him. The television was never on. Instead it was a parade of almost daily visitors, his brothers, his son, the priest, the nurse, the nurse's aide, the hospice volunteer, and neighbors.

John was never at a loss for words, a story, a task, or errand for the volunteer. He loved to challenge others, to argue, to question—it was part of what made him a successful owner of a pharmacy as he said "back in the days when a pharmacist had to know a little bit about a lot of things." His reminiscences were always pleasant and heart-warming. No regrets, no unfulfilled goals, a loving wife and extended family who he heard from in some way every day.

When I arrived for my weekly visit as a hospice volunteer John announced that we would have coffee made "the Italian way"—strong enough to catch and keep your attention. He insisted that I learn how to make it and serve it properly with biscotti. This was my first task upon arrival every Friday, and of course, to run an errand to get coffee when the supply was low. He loved Italian food and insisted his wife and I take him to his favorite restaurant for lunch.

One visit day he was not in his recliner when I arrived but in bed asleep. Congestive heart failure had won the battle for his energy. It was a day or two later his wife called to say, "Thanks for your friendship and support. We always appreciated your visits. John won't need a cane anymore."

The family worked as a system. They missed John, but he was with them in spirit. They handled the grief of loss as they had other trials, with lots of food and Italian coffee for the many family and friends who came to celebrate his life.

After the Angels Have Left

To paraphrase Ernest Hemmingway (Cohen 2008), death breaks every one and afterward many are strong at the broken places. A loss, such as a death, has a fracturing effect on a family, whether temporary or permanent. The effects of this fracture usually begin following the funeral or memorial service when face-to-face emotional support from others outside the family begin to diminish and survivors return to their usual obligations and responsibilities while their grieving is ongoing. As one grieving spouse expressed it, "it's the time when all the angels have left that you feel most alone and vulnerable."

All families need to grieve to cope with loss—it's human to do so. However, families and individuals cope differently. Some families and individuals seem to be "stronger" and show few outward signs of their loss, while other family members show their tears more readily and freely. Not all families or individuals need to call upon resources outside the family, but all should know about the availability of grief support groups should they be needed. Grieving has no timelines or boundaries.

Grieving involves a substantial investment in physical and emotional stamina in rebuilding and repairing family relationships. The loss of a family member or relative affects both the immediate and extended family in some way irrespective of the geographical, social, or emotional closeness of its members. There is usually a family member who is the leader, convener, or facilitator who initiates the rebuilding and repairing process. Unless, of course, that person is the deceased.

Not all deaths have equal importance to the family system. That is why the death of a family leader is especially traumatic. Death disrupts the family equilibrium and also its emotional relationships. Family members are replaceable as leaders, but not as persons. Both the functional role and emotional dependence of a family leader are key in how the family system will be restored and how successfully it will function. New leaders can emerge from tragedy and enable family systems to flourish or fail depending on the degree of cohesiveness of the system and the commitment of family members to the system's success. After the angels leave is when the good and bad family dynamics show themselves. Family legacies continue whether they are helpful or hurtful.

Families as a unit do not generally seek help for issues relating to a recent or past death. Usually intervention is sought for a problem in a family member or a specific relationship. Often the death of a family member is not mentioned as part of the problem. Issues around a deceased family member occur when the deceased member is idealized and not seen as a person with both strengths and weaknesses, or there are relationship issues that were not resolved with the deceased family member, or the facts surrounding the death are confused, or unreal. These issues can result in unresolved mourning and displaced negative feelings toward other family members.

Family vulnerability to dysfunction is especially high following a violent death from a suicide, homicide, accident, or being killed in a war, that is, a death caused by an external action. Unlike natural death from disease or old age, someone is responsible for a violent death; the family cannot rest until the death is explained and the perpetrator is identified and justice carried out.

The drama of violent death is commonly told as a story. The retelling of a violent death is important to survivors in finding the key to restoring themselves, yet through retelling the event the terror and end result remain the same. According to Rynearson (2001), a psychiatrist, the violent death of a loved one differs from other types of death because the physical presence of the deceased is gone and there is no further opportunity to connect, except through memories formed by retelling the violent event.

There are organized support groups to help family members share their grief and retell their story as well as lobby for legislative change. Some groups are peer-led and others are professionally-led, but both provide support for retelling stories and an opportunity to resolve intense trauma and grief. Indeed in many instances of violent death the stories are never complete and the responsible person(s) are not found and brought to justice, leaving many stories with incomplete answers and life-long wounds.

Lingering Loss

There is an anonymous quote that says "death and taxes may be certain, but we don't have to die every year." Yet, every loss is both unique and cumulative. The full impact of a death may never be known because loss is not a single event with time-limited effects. The effects of a death may linger for a lifetime. While some therapists may seek to help a client with "closure," the emotional dynamics of a previous loss cannot be separated from a current one.

The impact of a death involves the interplay of many factors such as its suddenness, the circumstances surrounding it, the age of the decedent and several related feelings including the common ones of anger, guilt and loneliness. The effects of a death are experienced differently as we move through the lifecycle being triggered by various circumstances and interactions with family, friends and others. In this way the impact of a death can have lingering effects, which vary with the personalities and situations of those affected. The pervasiveness of the effects of a death may or may not become fully apparent to others.

We express the personal impact of a loss through the process of grieving. Grieving may begin prior to the actual death of a person when he is told by a physician that he has a terminal illness and a caregiving plan needs to be developed. Grieving in this instance may extend for months, years, or even decades in the case of a chronic illness. On the other hand, a sudden infant death provides little or no warning and preparation for the parents. Grief behavior is personal and unique hence overt grief behavior is not always an accurate indication of how a person is coping with a loss.

Roxann joined a grief group shortly after her second husband died. She was having a difficult time with this loss as the marriage was not a happy one. She remarried a second time after her first husband's death. She was angry that her husband refused to change his life habits following a heart attack and she felt guilty for not being more assertive in getting him to change his habits. She initially felt guilty remarrying, especially since the second marriage was not a happy one. She blamed herself for not doing more to make her second marriage work. She grieved the loss of both of her husbands and experienced profound episodes of loneliness with the thought that she would not remarry again. Her grief spanned the 25 years of her two marriages.

Anger, guilt and loneliness are common emotions present in the grieving process. Anger is often vented on the decedent, oneself, and/or God. Guilt is focused around "what should or could have been done to prevent the death." And loneliness is expressed to elicit support and advice from others. Grief groups are one option to help grievers gain perspective from the insight and experiences of others. Some people avoid groups and prefer to grieve alone. The downside of this choice is that one can "become stuck in grief" by limiting their options. Feelings need to be expressed, and owned, and not hidden. It is through sharing our losses that we learn the value of time.

Multiple Loss

Loss does not occur in life in patterned or predictable ways. We sometimes experience several losses of differing magnitudes and types simultaneously; as the expression goes "when it rains it pours." There is a Polish saying, "misfortune walks in pairs." Multiple losses may tax the coping skills of a caregiver resulting in bereavement overload. Indeed, a loss that has not been fully grieved can resurface, adding to the risk of grief overload. Family caregivers may need the assistance of professional support.

References

Cohen, R. M. (2008). *Strong at the broken places: Voices of Illness, a chorus of hope*. New York: Harper Collins.

Kleinman, A. (2008). Catastrophe and caregiving: The failure of medicine as an art. *The Lancet, 371*(9606), 22–23.

Poulin, M. J., Brown, S. L., Ubel, P., Smith, D. M., Jankovic, A., & Langa, K. M. (2010). Does a helping hand mean a heavy heart? Helping behavior and well-being among spouse caregivers. *Psychology and Aging, 25*(1), 108–117.

Rynearson, E. K. (2001). *Retelling violent death*. New York: Routledge.

Span, P. (2014). Bounced from hospice. *The New York Times*, January 7, 2014.

Chapter 7
Healing Behavior for Caregivers

Abstract There are several behaviors that can facilitate adaptation to a terminal disease and the dying process. Connectedness with others, an interest area, goal or purpose for living, spiritual support, peace with the past, positive reflections on life satisfactions and accomplishments, leaving a legacy and gratitude for the gift of caregiving are ways that both surviving relatives and dying patients can help to soften survivors to have positive memories following the death. Time runs out differently for each one of us. While we do not control the timing of terminal disease and death, we can influence to some degree, how they affect the quality of our time living.

Keywords Assisted living · Connections · Long-term care · Self-help and support groups

Life-threatening illness interrupts and changes every aspect of our lives. There is no recipe for what to expect or how to cope. Frank (1991) has said there is no exemplary way to be ill. Our social connections with others and our value of time are unique to each of us.

Learning that one has a terminal disease should not be a shock as we all know that eventually everyone will experience death. However, learning that one has a terminal illness becomes a shock when we personalize the realization of loss. Time runs out differently for each one of us. For some it comes too early in life, for others it disrupts family and career at their prime, and for still others it is too emotionally and physically painful or incapacitating. While we do not control the timing of terminal disease and death, we can influence, to some degree, how they affect the quality of our time while living.

Time wounds us all. When we are wounded we grieve for what we value that has been changed. We react to being wounded differently. In the case of terminal illness the wound is permanent, but our reactions to it can be adaptive (Frank 1995).

There are several behaviors that can facilitate adaptation to a terminal disease and the dying process (Chentsova-Dutton et al. 2000).

J.G. Bruhn, *After Diagnosis: Family Caregiving with Hospice Patients*,
SpringerBriefs in Well-Being and Quality of Life Research,
DOI 10.1007/978-3-319-29803-0_7

1. *Connectedness with others.* It is not uncommon after a person learns they have a terminal illness to withdraw from other people including family. Withdrawal is often due to depression and feelings of hopelessness, which minimizes communication and involvement in activities. Of course, treatment interventions and their side effects can make the person sick and encourage their reduced social participation. As a terminal disease progresses the mobility of the ill person may be reduced also limiting their social interaction. Nonetheless, a person with a terminal illness needs to maintain their social skills to keep them connected with others. It is too easy for patients in some group homes and nursing homes to sit for hours in recliners in front of television until they are awakened for the next meal. Connectedness can involve visits from friends and volunteers, card games, sensory stimulation, cognitive activity such as reading books and magazines, and listening to books on tape, and walks around the home or facility. The positive effects of various interventions such as pet or music therapy are well known even for dementia patients.
2. *An interest area, goal or purpose for living.* Many people have interest areas, or hobbies which they often give up after they learn they have a terminal illness. Everyone needs a goal or purpose for living. When a person learns that they have a terminal illness it is easy to stop looking ahead and merely mark time waiting to die. Many group and nursing homes have organized activities to keep residents active and involved with others. Research has shown that people admitted to long-term care facilities have a high mortality the first year after admission. This has been called "life expectancy compression" (Orestis 2009). It is a high-risk period for emotional and social disconnectedness. A purpose for living, no matter how simplistic it may be, can sustain both physical and mental health.
3. *Spiritual support.* Most hospice, hospitals, and some rehabilitation centers and nursing homes provide access to chaplaincy services and offer weekly religious gatherings. In addition, many churches provide pastoral visits and care ministry outreach activities for their members when they become homebound or institution-bound. Some persons may not be religious, spiritual, or be affiliated with a religious denomination, but nonetheless they enjoy having conversations or reading books or magazines that inspire thoughtfulness and hope. For those who are believers in divine intervention, solo prayer or prayer groups are also meaningful and satisfying ways to maintain spiritual support.
4. *Peace with the past.* The combination of a terminal illness and increasing age can cause some people to dwell on their past life and become overwhelmed with regret, guilt, and disappointment. It is important to keep a positive, hopeful, and optimistic attitude to facilitate well-being, healing, and reinforce one's self concept (Groopman 2004). We all have made decisions or engaged in behavior that we regret, but we can make a truce with our past.

   We may benefit from the supportive environment of a self-help group and learn by sharing our story with others how common experiences unite us. Forgiveness is a great remedy for the hurts and failures of our earlier lives. A professor of psychiatry at one of the medical schools in the U.S. said that people ought to respect a person's right to die mad, with a frown instead of a smile (Kapp 2000).

His point is to allow people to remain true to their individual character and personality to the very end. Positive growth at the end of life should not be forced paternalistically on an unwilling patient anymore than an unwanted feeding tube or respirator. How "at peace" a dying patient feels about their life is a choice everyone is free to make.

5. *Reflections on life satisfactions and accomplishments*. Too often we don't ask the dying to talk about their satisfactions and accomplishments in life, but rather, the survivors talk about them after the fact in a memorial service. Sometimes dying persons are known most by their particular disorder rather than their distinguished persona. One reason dying persons need to "look back" is to savor and share their satisfactions and accomplishments. Every person is a potential mentor for someone else—sharing stories of success, hope, overcoming odds and obstacles, and challenges, is one way to positively engage dying persons in being hopeful about building on their legacies (Albom 1997).
6. *Leaving a legacy*. Everyone leaves a legacy of themselves. It can be a son or daughter that follows in their career footsteps, their modeling of giving back, or how they make a difference in the lives of others (Hartog 2012). Great people often leave simple legacies and simple, ordinary people often leave great legacies. What a person leaves undone for others to do after they are gone are stories that are often left untold, and hence, unfulfilled. Time permitting we need to enable the dying to share their legacies verbally and in writing before they pass.
7. *Gratitude for the gift of caregiving*. It has been said that time can be given as a gift. Caregiving is an example of such a gift. All terminally ill persons know that their lives are literally in the hands of caregivers, who, paid or volunteer, share their time with the dying person. Sometimes the dying person remains at home with the family providing as much care as within their expertise and resources; others find the needs of the dying person to be too demanding and admit the person to a facility providing the appropriate level of care; still others find that home care can be maintained with the help of caregivers such as hospice. Time spent with the sick and dying is a generous gift; it illustrates the importance of loving relationships and respect for their situations.

Sociologist Wuthnow (1991) has said that Americans need to learn better how to care for each other and to be motivated to put their good intentions into practice. Perhaps we could also learn how to be effective current and future caregivers. We could learn what constitutes effective caregiving by volunteering in facilities that provide various types of assisted and/or long-term care, enrolling in workshops on caregiving, accessing information on the internet, and sharing experiences with friends who have been caregivers to family members. We need to have more kindness in American life to mitigate social ills, humanize public policy, and ensure common human decency.

References

Albom, M. (1997). *Tuesdays with Morrie.* New York: Doubleday.

Chentsova-Dutton, Y., Shuchter, S., Hutchin, S., Strause, L., Burns, K., & Zisook, S. (2000). The psychological and physical health of hospice caregivers. *Annals of Clinical Psychiatry, 12*(1), 19–27.

Frank, A. W. (1991). *At the will of the body: Reflections on illness*. Boston: Houghton Mifflin Co.

Frank, A. W. (1995). *The wounded storyteller*. Chicago: University of Chicago Press.

Groopman, J. (2004). *The anatomy of hope*. New York: Random House.

Hartog, H. (2012). *Someday all this will be yours: A history of inheritance and old age*. Cambridge, MA. Harvard University Press.

Kapp, M. B. (2000). *The right to die mad* (pp. 10–11). Winter: The Pharos.

Orestis, C. (2009). Life expectancy compression: Effects on longevity after moving into an LTC facility. *Insurance News Net Magazine*, October 2009.

Wuthnow, R. (1991). *Acts of compassion: Caring for others and helping ourselves*. New York: Princeton University Press.

Chapter 8
Vignettes of Family Caregiving

Abstract This chapter presents several detailed examples of different situations of caregiving by family members, discussing the options available including limited finances and limited number of family members to provide care.

Keywords Elder transitions • Home health care service • Hospice volunteers • Long distance care

What to Do About Aunt Mary?

It was early December, 2007 when my sister and I (JGB) wrote to our Aunt Mary about arranging our annual Christmas visit. We usually flew from Phoenix to Northern California and rented a car to drive to where Aunt Mary had lived for over fifty years. She lived in the same house she had purchased new when she taught school in the area. Now retired for almost thirty years, she looked and acted much younger than her 98 years. She was the family's gatherer of news, pictures and made a point in keeping everyone connected. Her hand-written letters, often with newspaper clippings of stories or philosophy, could be counted on as regular as the church newsletter. We had made Christmas a time to spend with Aunt Mary as she lived alone and as the years left their limitations on her she found it difficult to travel to see her younger sisters and nieces and nephews and their children. Family visited Aunt Mary, but not often enough in our opinion. Holidays were special for families, and we chose to accept Aunt Mary's open invitation to visit. And we enjoyed our visits as Aunt Mary was a card player, puzzle solver, a witty storyteller, who enjoyed eating out, seeing the decorated homes at Christmas, and a fan of music and theater. We left our visits with Aunt Mary with sadness about their shortness and we felt uplifted and energized and grew in our love and respect for her.

We were surprised, therefore, not to receive any response to our letter to her; she was always so conscientious! We wondered about her well-being so we called her. "Why, of course," she said, she welcomed us and we agreed to arrive a few days

J.G. Bruhn, *After Diagnosis: Family Caregiving with Hospice Patients*,
SpringerBriefs in Well-Being and Quality of Life Research,
DOI 10.1007/978-3-319-29803-0_8

before December 24th and stay until New Years. Her voice sounded a bit weak, but after all she was 98 years old.

We arrived at Aunt Mary's house about mid-afternoon. The morning paper was still on the doorstep, unusual because Aunt Mary worked all the available puzzles in the morning paper every day after breakfast. It took some time after the doorbell and knocks on the door before Aunt Mary came to the door with her walker. She looked frail and thin and gave us tentative hugs so as not to lose her balance. We spent the evening catching up on family news and after a small snack, Mary excused herself and retired to her bedroom. We were surprised; she was always a conversationalist.

We noticed a pile of mail at one end of the kitchen table, a refrigerator that needed restocking, and the guest beds unprepared for us as they were in previous visits. It was 10:00 a.m. the next day, after my sister and I had breakfast, that we decided to knock on Aunt Mary's bedroom door. She had always prepared breakfast for all of us before or suggested a visit to a local restaurant. It took about an hour for Aunt Mary to get ready for the day. We asked her about getting to the grocery store, the pile of mail, and getting to her hair and doctor's appointments. Indeed, she had been driving her 1966 Chevy Malibu to run errands, play bridge with friends, and maintain her appointments. While we were there we used the rental car which I drove as Aunt Mary occupied the front seat to give directions and cautions. I felt unsafe just thinking about how she managed to drive her car with her degree of frailty and general alertness. After two days at Aunt Mary's my sister and I took a long walk in the neighborhood to discuss "What do we do about Aunt Mary?"

One of our biggest concerns was Aunt Mary's safety. While she lived in a cul de sac with neighbors who monitored each other's activities, the larger neighborhood had deteriorated and the residents more temporary. We knew Aunt Mary was adamant about staying in her house as she had turned down previous suggestions we had made about moving to an apartment or to live with one of us in Phoenix. Indeed, her friends were all in the Sacramento area and weekly bridge had become the centerpiece of their social network. We discussed options to present to Aunt Mary, which included assisted living or getting a roommate to live with her. We had done some homework and heard of a local health care group called the Angels of Mercy, which provided a variety of services in one's home on a daily or weekly basis. This option seemed to be the best one we thought as it respected Aunt Mary's autonomy, and was affordable. At least it was a first step given the shortness of our visit and it being a major holiday season. We presented our concern about safety to Aunt Mary when she awakened from a nap of several hours. We called Angels of Mercy and the owner came to Aunt Mary's house within the hour to meet Mary and discuss our needs and possible arrangements. We agreed that a nurse's aide would visit Aunt Mary three times a week, do minor house cleaning, laundry, prepare lunch, and be a friend for four hours each visit. The plan was put in place the week after Christmas.

Angels of Mercy would inform me by email of how Aunt Mary was doing and any problems. I, too, would call Aunt Mary to get her opinion about this arrangement. Initially the Angels of Mercy had to work out some issues related to time, tasks, and authority, but overall things worked well. I planned on returning at least once a month.

There were several other issues besides safety that had to be addressed before we returned to Phoenix. One was the pile of mail on the kitchen table. When I asked Aunt Mary about the mail she said, "I didn't know what to do with it so I put it in a pile on the table." Not surprisingly bills had not been paid for several months and had grown substantially with late fees, and with repeated threats to cut off service. We learned from the yardman that electric service had been cut off and following her call to the yardman to inform him, he had paid the bill. Similar threats existed for water and phone services. The yardman had asked Aunt Mary about any relatives at the time and Aunt Mary said that she had none. I sorted the mail, paid the bills before we returned to Phoenix and informed Aunt Mary that I would have her mail forwarded to me and I would make out the checks for her to sign and mail. The biggest problem was what to do to get her multiple magazine subscriptions cancelled. She had been an easy target for magazine vendors for years.

Another issue we needed to address was Aunt Mary's ability to drive her car. She talked about her car as if it were her child. The car was a 1966 vintage model, Chevrolet with less than 100,000 miles, with the original paint and pampered; oil was changed religiously every 5,000 miles and recorded in a journal kept in the glove box. The car drew many offers from young men when Aunt Mary filled up with gas at her usual gas station. In Aunt Mary's eyes the car and she were inseparable, and was worth at least $20,000! But, after seeing Aunt Mary's dependence on a walker and her slow reaction time while driving, I feared for her life and those lives of others, especially children near school zones. Even though we discussed her responsibilities as a car owner, several times heatedly, she said that she was going to continue to drive. She was not going to ask others for rides! And, besides how would she get to contract bridge each week to see her fellow card players who lived in a local nursing home if she couldn't drive? This problem could not be resolved during our Christmas visit, but I knew it would sneak up and bite us again, which it did.

Still another major issue to be addressed before we left for Phoenix was Aunt Mary's health care. Aunt Mary had been blessed with good health during her lifetime needing only doctor visits for allergy shots. But, she never talked about her health; she never complained about aches and pains. She was not into cooking or following a balanced diet. This was apparent to us in her loss of weight and strength. We stressed with Angels of Mercy the importance of getting her to buy more fresh fruit and vegetables on visits to the grocery store. However, Aunt Mary's attitudes and habits were not easily changed. She was seeing a doctor and on medications for osteoarthritis; the doctor also referred her for physical therapy and nutritional services. We left feeling good about Aunt Mary's health care even though her ability to follow through was less than we hoped for.

It's now 2008 and we are back in Phoenix. I kept in touch with the Angels of Mercy and also Aunt Mary. In February we celebrated Aunt Mary's 99th birthday. We talked about making it to 100. She said the neighbors were planning to have a party for her then. The arrangements with the Angels of Mercy were working well except there were some changes in the nurse's aides causing some schedule changes and Aunt Mary would not let the aides prepare her meals. Instead Aunt Mary and the aide went to Mary's favorite sandwich shop where she could get homemade ice cream for dessert. And yes, despite my continuing objections, Aunt Mary was driving her car when I was not there.

In April I received a call from Angels of Mercy saying that Aunt Mary was hospitalized for dizziness, weakness and dehydration. I returned to California. I found her sitting up in bed holding forth with several nurses who were surprised to see me as Aunt Mary had told them she had no living family members. The doctor told me to watch for falls and gave me a prescription. I took Aunt Mary home. She had a follow-up visit with her usual doctor a week later. I took her to that appointment. The doctor told Aunt Mary and me that she should be in an assisted living facility; he was concerned about her poor nutrition and risk of falling. Aunt Mary smiled politely. She was opposed to moving to a facility. I did some research on available, affordable assisted living facilities in the area. Meanwhile Aunt Mary agreed to increasing the coverage by the Angels of Mercy to five hours a day five days a week. I returned to Phoenix.

In June I returned to visit Aunt Mary and convinced her to visit three assisted living facilities that were within her budget. She was on a modest teacher's retirement plan. Aunt Mary never voiced an opinion about the facilities and it didn't matter because I later discovered that her health insurance would not help pay for assisted living, only nursing home care. So we settled for as much care from Angels of Mercy as she could afford. I continued to worry about falls and her well-being over weekends. She seemed to be accepting of more visits by the Angels of Mercy as long as she could stay in her home.

I had been back in Phoenix for about a month when I received a call from Angels of Mercy alerting me that, in their opinion, Aunt Mary needed assisted living as she was becoming more frail and stubborn about doing what she wanted to do without asking for help. For some reason she felt more comfortable calling the yardman for help than her neighbors or the Angels of Mercy. This is precisely who she called when she returned from an appointment to find her house had been burglarized. The yardman called me and the police. I quickly arranged a trip to California.

While her house was ransacked it was apparent the thieves knew what they wanted and cleaned out her jewelry in an adjacent bedroom and blank checks from her desk in her bedroom. The thieves had a plan to carry out the robbery during a two-hour block of time when she would be at a doctor's appointment. They had gained entrance through the unlocked side door to the garage and lifted the door entering the family room from the garage off of its hinges to enter the house. It looked like a plan that was developed knowing Aunt Mary's schedule as she was at home most of the time. Aunt Mary's reaction to the loss of her jewelry was almost one of disinterest, stating that most of it was inexpensive costume jewelry. I returned to Phoenix after talking with the police and insurance adjuster.

In August I received a call from the Angels of Mercy to say that Aunt Mary was in a car accident, but unhurt. I called her at home. She minimized the accident not recalling how it happened. She was returning home when she said she heard a noise but kept on driving. When she pulled into her driveway she had two shredded tires on the right side of the car and some minor scratches. Her neighbor, who worked for a tire business, replaced the tires for her. And that was the end of her story. At my next visit a few weeks later I sat down with Aunt Mary eye-to-eye and asked for her car keys. She refused despite my examples of how she as a former school teacher was putting school children at the nearby school at risk, she refused to discuss giving up the car. It was then that I realized that I was trying to be rational with someone who wasn't. That night, before I was to return to Phoenix, I removed her car keys from her purse and informed the Angels of Mercy to take her wherever she needed to go, which they did. I knew, however, that Aunt Mary did not stop driving. Her neighbor said she told him, "He (referring to me) doesn't know I have another key!" We never discussed the topic again, although it was always on my mind.

The morning of October 30, 2008 I received a call from the Angels of Mercy that the nurse's aide found Aunt Mary in the bathtub, her body was warm, but there was no pulse. The EMTs attempted resuscitation unsuccessfully. Aunt Mary had died peacefully in her own home alone as she would have wanted, but disappointed that she didn't reach 100! I knew what to do about Aunt Mary. We had made arrangements for her at a funeral home and cemetery on one of my visits to California. It was also where many of her friends were buried. She had the last say in where she wanted to be.

My later reflections on my care of Aunt Mary included the impact of her progressive dementia on her and on me, emotionally and physically. We were both emotionally drained and had neglected our physical health. First, for a person as fiercely independent who strived to be proactive and in control, the advent of dementia symptoms must have been devastating to Aunt Mary, but she kept her fears to herself. The first clue that something was wrong was losing control over her handwriting. Her checkbook reflected this change. And, it explains why she was overwhelmed by the mail, especially the bills which needed checks to be mailed. The first clue to me that something was wrong was the abrupt termination of her letters, always frequent and carefully written. I was in denial of the fact that Aunt Mary had dementia as I recalled her lucid times and always perceived her "in charge" of her life. Also, being recently retired I could envision myself in the same predicament. She was one of my favorite aunts as we had a lot of academic, social, and community interests in common. Rarely did she complain about anything—she always looked the same to me.

Aunt Mary should have been in an assisted living facility, but she was so opposed to the idea of leaving and selling her home that doing that against her will would have been cowardly and certain to be a cause of her death. Had she survived I was going to ask her doctor about at home hospice care. It would have meant that Aunt Mary would have had to accept the fact that she might not live to be 100. But, the Angels of Mercy organization served both Aunt Mary and me, as a geographically remote caregiver, well. We were blessed that Aunt Mary did not experience a fall, a stroke, or a disabling car accident. She did, in fact, have a legion of Angels who provided preventive care to a stubborn, but loving, lady who appreciated them all.

Good Transitions for a Determined Dad

It was a daily routine; Robert would take a nap in his favorite chair while his wife would do exercises in her nearby favorite room. One evening Robert awoke, startled by silence, to find his wife of over 50 years, Eileen, stretched out on the floor and not breathing. Although Eileen's sudden death was a great shock to Robert, she left a legacy, a journal and calendar of her everyday activities and the names and addresses of friends to whom she sent cards. Robert was determined to continue her legacy, and used her journal and calendars to map out his life and continue the card tradition after her death. She began every day with prayer and exercise and that is how Robert began his day for years to come. The practice of a daily routine fit Robert's occupation as the owner of a maintenance business servicing malls and shopping areas. He was a collector of "things" that he thought might be useful to him in the future. His backyard was filled with small sheds containing the things he collected, but rarely used, because he could not find them in the constantly growing and overwhelming inventory. Robert was a saver, a collector of things and memories, and also grew attached to Nipper, a cockatiel who became a beloved companion for over 27 years.

Robert was a quiet, unassuming person, who seemed to anticipate life and was never a burden to others. Robert always enjoyed a good meal, saying with a smile on his face that he loved all kinds of food and lots of it! A year after Eileen's death he decided to move to the Southwest to be closer to one of his sons and his family. This was an enormous transition, as he had been in the same house for over 30 years, and his massive collection of "useful things" had to be sold, donated or tossed away. He was determined to make the transition, so that he could spend more time with his son's family and especially his two granddaughters who were the lights of his life. First he chose an apartment within a senior community about 30 min from his son's home. After some time he and his family realized he needed more help with weekly activities, so he moved to an apartment about five minutes from his son's house. Robert always became well known wherever he lived, making the effort to meet new people and never turning down an opportunity to have a cup of coffee and talk about his family, his church, his career, World War II or any other topic that might come up.

His car was important to him to get to early morning church services on Sunday. He would often arrive two hours before services and sit in his car drinking coffee and reading the Sunday paper until his family arrived for services. He enjoyed a simple and routine life style. He loved Sunday brunch and Friday nights were favorite times to join his family for a meal.

But as the years passed, Robert became a less astute driver and his son was not looking forward to talking with his dad about giving up his car. To his son's surprise, Robert decided, without discussion, to give his car to his oldest granddaughter who recently got her driver's license and would be starting college. Robert acquired a motorized cart to do his shopping. He became a familiar sight in the neighborhood with his cart's long antenna and flag to announce his presence. Robert was well known by neighbors and shop keepers who kept an eye out for him as he traveled many blocks from home, usually to join friends for coffee or stock up on his supply of greeting cards. Robert's family was often taken aside by people they didn't know who told them of his good humor, positive attitude and smile that often made their days.

Robert was an avid reader and loved to watch baseball and football games, especially his San Diego Chargers and Padres. Over the next few years Robert's hearing was barely helped by his hearing aids. He developed macular degeneration, and began losing sight. He needed help daily, and between his family and a few hours of in-home nursing care, he managed on his own for a while more.

Robert was experiencing increased problems with his hearing and sight, and despite a life of mostly good health, there were issues of concern about his mobility, falling and arterial disease. His son discussed the possibility of an assisted living facility which Robert accepted willingly. While watching his favorite sports on television or reading his Bible, which he kept on a nearby table, became infrequent, he seemed content to be present with others in the common room. Robert could often be seen in his favorite spot at the entrance of the assisted living facility where he greeted visitors and engaged with staff. He looked forward to visits from the clergy and his son and family, especially his two granddaughters. As always, he enjoyed the food. He was kind to the wait staff and was often treated to double desserts and lots of coffee. Many residents complained incessantly and treated the staff with disdain. Robert would tell his family that he avoided the complainers and could not understand why they always looked for problems rather than finding the good that existed. Robert made great friends with a man named Will whom he shared most of his meals with. Will would arrive early, prepare their table and have Robert's hot coffee waiting when he arrived. Will would also order Robert's favorite meals for him and would always make sure that the kitchen staff gave Robert extra food. Robert enjoyed the activities and the people and was in fact, a sought after dancer at the Valentine's Dance. He was famous for his "thumbs up" sign to everyone; even when he became almost totally deaf, blind, and wheelchair bound, he would stick his thumb up when he was aware of a friend nearby. He and Nipper transitioned well to assisted living and its many levels of care. Robert and Nipper would receive extra visits from staff and neighbors who came by to hear Nipper's diatribe of "Pretty Bird" and "Nipper, Nipper, Nipper."

As he neared his 90th birthday the early signs of dementia set in requiring the need to move Robert to a facility with a Memory Care Unit. So Robert and Nipper moved again without complaint. But Robert acquired a new friend; a Chihuahua named "Minnie," the pet of one of the caregivers, who usually could be found in Robert's lap, giving him kisses on his neck. Everyone liked Robert and even though his communication was now greatly limited, he would often give a quick smile or a thumbs up. Robert always was a determined individual who had a positive outlook on life, no matter what the circumstances were. Robert was driven by his faith, his love of family and country, the legacy left by his wife and the assurance that they would be together again. One day Robert's longtime companion Nipper was found at the bottom of his cage. Within a few months Robert stopped eating and died peacefully, much the way he lived his life.

Being Present Was Enough

Hi Bill! I'm John. As he looked at me his eyes were vacuous. He was sitting at the kitchen table in a generous bathrobe, barefooted, his face camouflaged by several days of beard growth, irritated by an oxygen tube that limited his freedom. He didn't get up. He didn't extend a hand. He was without words. He looked empty.

His wife introduced me as a hospice volunteer who would stay with him for the next three hours once a week for the forthcoming weeks so she could experience respite. His wife showed me his prepared lunch in the refrigerator and told me that following lunch he always took a lengthy nap. He knew where his medications were and when to take them. She left her cell phone number in case of an emergency and said goodbye.

As the door closed Bill looked at me across the kitchen table and said, "And what will you do?" "I'm here as a friend and support person," I said. "I have no friends," he said, and "I don't need anything." As the afternoon passed we were in a dialogue that lasted well past Bill's usual lunch time and nap time. What had initially appeared to be Bill's emptiness was his aloneness. He was one of those types who offer help to others, but do not ask for it. And being self-effacing, with a twinge of sarcasm and dry humor, Bill did not easily ask for help from others. Indeed, being a friend to Bill was an initiation process which was not appealing to many. So Bill's wife was also his best friend.

Bill had been "on empty" before in his life but was a survivor until his last doctor's appointment where he once again experienced aloneness. He had heard the doctor's first and last words but nothing in between. "You need to get your affairs in order… maybe six months more." Hospice was an unknown to Bill, but he was concerned about his doting wife and her need for respite from him. And, while hospice didn't make promises he liked being at home and the realistic attitude of the personnel. They were his friends and advocates and his care was the focus of attention. His sarcasm and dry humor were occasionally offensive to his caregivers but he apologized. He was accepted for who he was. What better friends could one have?

Bill didn't share who he was easily. He was a survivor of a plane crash. He was a survivor of lung cancer. He was a millionaire with only a high school education. He was used to being self-reliant. Friends needed him. So being told that his journey with COPD and failing eyesight and hearing would be physically painless, this was a prognosis for which he didn't need a friend. He felt he could survive without friends, but he discovered that friends found him. Bill confided that he had no unmet hopes or dreams. He had travelled, was successful in business, had a good family, and enjoyed steak, ice cream, card games, and gambling. He died peacefully in bed. His wife said that he always looked forward to visits from his hospice friends. At each visit he escorted me to the door, smiled, and thanked me for coming. Being present was enough.

Separate yet Together

Betty and Fred were inseparable for 68 years. Never did they expect that in their final years they would be living down the hall from one another in the same group home. Neither one of them expected to live as long as they did. Betty was the professional and Fred was the salesman. Both were devoted to one another while strongly defending their independent interests—for Betty it was talking about nutrition and the world of academics, for Fred it was sports. Ironically when Betty became blind she listened to tapes and CDs, when Fred became hard of hearing he read sports magazines and set the TV on his favorite sports channel. They were only a shout across the hall when they needed each other and had daily meals together with the other residents. And, they worried about each other.

Betty and Fred also lived longer than their step-daughter expected. Betty and Fred's retirement savings were being depleted. So, much to the disappointment of Betty and Fred, their step-daughter moved Fred to her home under her care. But Fred's unsteady gait led to a fall and broken arm while the daughter was at work. After a few weeks Fred was moved back to his former room at the group home. However, the step-daughter caused a family riff by discussing finances that left Betty and Fred feeling guilty that they were living so long and the possible future costs to their daughter. The daughter visited less often and, except for visits from a few of their friends who were still able and mobile, they were left to pass the time with activities at the group home. A son had not been heard from in years and Betty and Fred did not know his whereabouts.

Over a few months Betty lost her appetite and consequently weight and her stamina. She was placed under hospice care and kept more to herself, saying that she did not feel well. One morning Fred discovered Betty dead in bed. Profoundly sad, Fred was not his usual self as he said, "We had 68 wonderful years together—I am glad she was my wife."

It has been almost two years since Betty passed. Fred will soon celebrate his 95th birthday. Only recently as his cane no longer provided enough stability, had he been asked to use the wheelchair and his memory is slipping. He spends his days in a large recliner dozing off while watching sports on TV and reading Sports Illustrated. "I don't know what we would do without sports," he says. He tries to get out of his chair to welcome a visitor only succeeding on the third attempt, but his always ready smile and firm handshake make a person feel that Fred is a life-long friend who is eager to see you. He is always ready to talk about his days in the Air Force during WWII and his early days as a football player. As he looks up at the photos on the wall facing him he is gracious about his memories of Betty and how he is lucky that she married him. And across the hall, in Betty's former room, is a patient with dementia, unable to connect with Fred. Fred no longer has to shout; he feels his memories in his heart.

Do You Love Me?

The family caregiver needs love, too. As Maria prepared to leave for a few hours of respite she bent over her bedridden husband and asked, "Do you love me?" On lucid days the patient would whisper "Yes," and on other days the patient didn't acknowledge the question. Maria felt guilty taking respite time twice weekly during which time hospice provided a volunteer to watch over her husband. Maria spent most all of the hours during the day sitting in a chair beside her husband's bed, tending to his every need. Sometimes her husband would stay awake at night, unable to sleep because he had slept all day. Maria adapted to his schedule. Maria's own self-care was minimal on days when her husband experienced frustration, pain, or anger and she felt that his needs were primary over hers.

A "Yes" answer to the question "Do you love me?" helped to reassure Maria that providing 24 h care for her husband for the past two years was what she needed to hear to keep going. A stroke and dementia had compromised his cognitive and movement skills, and limited his conversation. Sometimes her husband was verbally abusive or spit out his medication, behaviors that Maria took to heart. Repeating the question "Do you love me?" therefore, was asked with tentativeness and mixed expectations of how her husband would respond.

As the patient had difficulty swallowing, he ate less and progressively lost weight, weakening his large stature. His weakened voice became a whisper and reduced conversations to expressing immediate needs for medication, liquids, and toileting. When lucid the patient's answer to the question "Do you love me?" became a nod of the head and a faint smile. Maria responded with a kiss and a sigh.

Chapter 9
Renewal and Remembrances

Abstract There is a downside to caregiving and that is burnout. It is not unexpected that caregivers may experience new or renewed health problems of their own. Compassion fatigue is a type of burnout characterized by a gradual lessening of compassion over time. Some level of burnout can be expected in every person who has served as a caregiver even for a short time. There are a variety of options for family caregivers to become renewed following their time of caregiving. One of the more common feelings experienced after a period of caregiving is loneliness. Every caregiver's situation is unique, but self-care is an essential part of a caregiver's renewal. Hospice attempts to create a balance in the life of the soon-to-die and their survivors by recognizing and sharing the good in each other's lives.

Keywords Grief groups · Health of caregivers · Resolving differences · Trauma in caregivers

Caregiving takes enormous energy—physical, mental, and spiritual. The energy expended in giving care to the dying is compounded by the length of time a person needing care lives, the quality of their decline as related to pain and suffering, and their ability to respond to their environment and to interact with those giving care (Figley 1995).

There is a downside to caregiving and that is burnout. Burnout is not simply working long hours. It involves the compression of several emotions including depression, fatigue, cynicism, disillusionment, helplessness, and self–doubts about their competence and the value of their caregiving efforts (Navaie-Waliser et al. 2002). Caregivers are sometimes reluctant to express those feelings to others, especially when caregiving for a family member. Therefore, it is not unexpected that caregivers may experience new or renewed health problems of their own.

Compassion fatigue is a type of burnout (Abendroth and Flannery 2006). It is characterized by a gradual lessening of compassion over time. Persons who are most likely to be at risk for developing compassion fatigue are those people who have traits valued in caregiving such as being conscientious, self-giving, and who have high levels of stress and low levels of social support in their own lives. Showing

J.G. Bruhn, *After Diagnosis: Family Caregiving with Hospice Patients*,
SpringerBriefs in Well-Being and Quality of Life Research,
DOI 10.1007/978-3-319-29803-0_9

compassion for someone whose suffering is continuous or unresolvable can further tax the nature of a compassionate caregiver, sometimes leading to abusive behavior.

Some level of burnout can be expected in every person who has served as a caregiver to a deceased family member even for a short time. Many family members fail to realize how demanding caregiving is, especially if one member of the family is doing the caregiving. At first most caregivers accept their role as caregivers with idealism, hope, and an eagerness to do well. Yet, caregiver burnout and/or compassion fatigue is a common feeling among caregivers. Caregivers find that serving their deceased family member includes many post-death responsibilities. Every caregiver needs a period of respite and renewal following the death of their loved one.

There are a variety of options for family caregivers to become renewed following their time of caregiving. One option is to join a grief support group, often sponsored by hospitals, churches, or hospices. These groups meet for varying lengths of time, and free of charge, and are ways to regain one's identity through the interaction of supportive peers. Usually family caregivers have devoted so much time to caregiving that they have become disconnected from their own networks. Joining a grief support group is a way to reconnect with others who have recently experienced a period of caregiving and loss (Volandes 2015).

Often caregivers give up living their own lives while being a caregiver to another person. Caregivers have a need to re-establish a routine of care for themselves regarding preventive health interventions from getting check-ups on their own physical and mental health. A plan to monitor one's own health is very important (Turner 2014).

One of the more common feelings experienced after a period of caregiving for a deceased family member is loneliness (Cacioppo and Patrick 2008). Loneliness is something over which we can exercise a certain degree of control. Loneliness has health consequences so it is important to seek out levels of connections that will help us re-establish our identity and develop personal goals. We all have a need for others not just in an abstract sense, but in groups and communities. Every caregiver's situation is unique, medically, emotionally and spiritually, but self-care is an essential part of a caregiver's renewal (Kearney et al. 2009).

Robinson-Whelen et al. (2001) found that, while former caregivers experienced some decrease in stress and negative affect after caregiving, they maintained a high degree of depression and loneliness, and in fact psychologically they were similar to current caregivers. Caregiving may, therefore, have long-term consequences for caregivers. It appears that caregivers who ruminated more about caregiving after bereavement reported more depression, stress, and greater social isolation (Bodnar and Kiecolt-Glaser 1994).

Helping valued loved ones may promote caregivers' well-being, although being a full-time caregiver can also present a serious threat to quality of life (Poulin et al. 2010). Caregivers who protect their own vulnerabilities and practice self-care are more likely to view caregiving as an opportunity to grow and experience positive emotions.

There are techniques available for caregivers to periodically self-assess the degree to which they are suffering trauma from their role as a caregiver. Pearlman and

Saakvitne (1996) have developed an instrument to be used by a wide variety of professionals and paraprofessionals that describes feelings, beliefs, and procedures that, if not balanced with positive actions, can lead to burnout or compassion fatigue. Learning new skills for improving emotional and psychological well-being can be a powerful preventive to make caregiving a positive and rewarding experience. Building social networks online and/or in person are essential in caring and coping throughout the caregiving process (Cross and Parker 2004).

Memories with Smiles

Whenever I dust my dresser I smile as I move the family photographs and recall the stories of three generations of family members. It takes a while to dust each picture and say a few words of love. The words are ones that could only be said after years of reflections on events, interactions, and remembrances. What is so impressive is that they all get along so well crowded together on top of the dresser!

It is amazing the words we think but never say at key times in our lives like the dying process of a family member, or after death at a memorial service, or on our national memorial day of remembrance. There is often so much emotion in us that we don't want to express, even after a loved one is gone. One of the ways often suggested to help the grieving with dealing with their grief is to memorialize the person through a scrapbook, poetry, art, a named scholarship, or other expressions, to make the continuity of life lost through death continue through happy remembrances. Eventually seeing a deceased family member's picture will bring on tears of happiness that one can still share the presence of their spirit rather than generate feelings of loss, regret, and even unresolved anger. Children, especially, should learn what a parent was, not what the parent could have been.

Learning that a person has six months or less to live elicits a variety of emotions from different people. Hospice attempts to create a balance in the life of the soon to die and their survivors by recognizing and sharing the good in each other's lives. Hospice helps to reduce social pain, which is the pain that we humans create by our actions and inaction. Physical pain can be controlled; spiritual pain can be healed; social pain can be ameliorated by forgiveness. Too often pride, stubbornness, or revenge prevent us from healing ourselves and others through forgiving words. It's never too late to ask for forgiveness. Memories too frequently suppress smiles and remember frowns. One of the ways to make sure that the family pictures on your dresser bring a smile to your face is to express your feelings about one another while still alive and people get a chance to love back.

References

Abendroth, M., & Flannery, J. (2006). Predicting the risk of compassion fatigue: A study of hospice nurses. *Journal of Hospice and Palliative Nursing, 8*(6), 346–356.

Bodnar, J. C., & Kiecolt-Glasser, J. K. (1994). Caregiver depression after bereavement: Chronic stress isn't over when it's over. *Psychology and Aging, 9*(3), 372–380.

Cacioppo, J. T., & Patrick, W. (2008). *Loneliness*. New York: W. W. Norton.

Cross, R., & Parker, A. (2004). *The hidden power of social networks*. Boston: Harvard Business School Publications Corporation.

Figley, C. R. (Ed.). (1995). *Compassion fatigue: Coping with secondary traumatic stress disorder in those who treat the traumatized*. New York: Brunner-Routledge.

Kearney, M. K., Weininger, R. B., Vachon, M. L. S., Harrison, R. L., & Mount, B. M. (2009). Self-care of physicians caring for patients at the end of life: Being connected...a key to my survival. *Journal of the American Medical Association, 301*(1), 1155–1164.

Navaie-Waliser, M., Feldman, P. H., Gould, D. A., Levine, C., Kuerbis, A. N., & Donelan, K. (2002). When the caregiver needs care: The plight of vulnerable caregivers. *American Journal of Public Health, 92*(3), 409–413.

Pearlman, L. A., & Saakvitne, K. W. (1996). *Transforming the pain: A workbook for vicarious traumatization*. New York: W. W. Norton & Co.

Poulin, M. J., Brown, S. L., Ubel, P., Smith, D. M., Jankovic, A., & Langa, K. M. (2010). Does a helping hand mean a heavy heart? Helping behavior and well-being among spouse caregivers. *Psychology and Aging, 25*(1), 108–117.

Robinson-Whelen, S., Tada, Y., MacCallum, R. C., McGuire, L., & Kiecolt-Glaser, J. K. (2001). Long-term caregiving: What happens when it ends? *Journal of Abnormal Psychology, 110*(4), 573–584.

Turner, J. (2014). Caregiving at life's end: Facing the challenges. American Hospice Foundation. Retrieved September 17, 2014. http://americanhospice.org/caregiving/caregiving-at-lifes-end-facing-the-challenges.

Volandes, A. E. (2015). *The conversation. A revolutionary plan for end-of-life care*. New York: Bloomsbury.

MIX
Papier aus verantwortungsvollen Quellen
Paper from responsible sources
FSC® C105338

If you have any concerns about our products,
you can contact us on
ProductSafety@springernature.com

In case Publisher is established outside the EU,
the EU authorized representative is:
Springer Nature Customer Service Center GmbH
Europaplatz 3, 69115 Heidelberg, Germany

Printed by Libri Plureos GmbH
in Hamburg, Germany